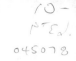

First Responder
Exam Preparation and Review

Daniel Limmer
Bob Elling

BRADY
Prentice Hall
Upper Saddle River, New Jersey 07458

Publisher: *Susan Katz*
Marketing manager: *Judy Streger*
Director of production and manufacturing: *Bruce Johnson*
Managing production editor: *Pat Walsh*
Senior production manager: *Ilene Sanford*
Editorial/production supervision: *Julie Boddorf*
Interior design/page layout: *Julie Boddorf*
Cover design: *Marianne Frasco*
Printer/binder: *Banta Company, Harrisonburg, VA*

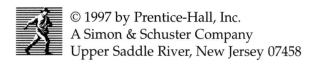

© 1997 by Prentice-Hall, Inc.
A Simon & Schuster Company
Upper Saddle River, New Jersey 07458

Printed in the United States of America
10 9 8 7 6 5 4 3 2 1

ISBN 0-8359-5021-2

Prentice-Hall International (UK) Limited, *London*
Prentice-Hall of Australia Pty. Limited, *Sydney*
Prentice-Hall Canada, Inc., *Toronto*
Prentice-Hall Hispanoamericana, S.A., *Mexico*
Prentice-Hall of India Private Limited, *New Delhi*
Prentice-Hall of Japan, Inc., *Tokyo*
Simon & Schuster Asia Pte. Ltd., *Singapore*
Editora Prentice-Hall do Brasil, Ltda., *Rio de Janeiro*

To Sarah Katherine, my little miss magic.

D. L.

To Kirsten, Laura, and Caitlin,
who continue to give me the strength
to jump the highest hurdles of life!

B. E.

Contents

Preface

Thank you for purchasing *First Responder Exam Preparation and Review.* This book takes a slightly different approach to exam preparation. This is due, in part to the new U.S. Department of Transportation National Standard First Responder Curriculum. Many of you are taking your initial First Responder training while others are recertifying or learning the new curriculum. This new curriculum changes the way many First Responders practice and makes a review book based on this new curriculum important.

Another important event which helped us decide to write this book is the National Registry of Emergency Medical Technicians' decision to offer national registry at the First Responder level. This is currently offered to EMT-Basics, EMT-Intermediates, and EMT-Paramedics. This is an important step for the First Responder level of certification. If you are preparing to take the National Registry exam we applaud you.

Most of this review book's chapters directly correlate with a lesson in the First Responder curriculum. Each chapter is broken down into four sections:

1. The chapter begins with a list of the First Responder curriculum objectives. Since most exams are based on the objectives, this will help you to identify the major themes of each lesson and determine your strengths and weaknesses in the lesson.

2. A quick review provides a brief discussion of the lesson's objectives. This review is short and to the point. It is designed to do just what the name implies: provide a quick review. It is

not a substitute for classroom or hands-on training. Try not to read the quick review immediately before taking the multiple choice questions as this may provide a grade on the lesson which does not reflect your true knowledge.

3. Each chapter has at least 15 multiple choice questions. The actual number of questions depends on the number of objectives in the corresponding lesson of the First Responder curriculum. The questions are in multiple choice format, similar to what you will see on national and state certification exams.

4. Answers *and* rationale are provided for all of the multiple choice questions. This provides the correct answer and *why* it is correct to help you understand and retain the information.

Due to the nature of the First Responder level of certification, agencies, regions, and states may add material to the curriculum. Therefore we have added optional information in the final chapters of the book. Since this does not correlate to the First Responder curriculum there are no objectives to refer to. The questions were based on common elements that are frequently added to the curriculum. Topics included in the optional information include medical emergencies not covered in the curriculum, automated external defibrillation, and oxygen administration.

We hope that this book helps you prepare for your classroom, certification, or National Registry examinations. We wish you luck on your examination as well as safety and enjoyment as you begin your experience as a First Responder. Remember the attributes of the First Responder as you begin or continue your First Responder responsibilities. It is always necessary to strive for quality patient care!

We welcome comments on the review manual. Your comments may be sent to:

Brady
Judy Streger, Marketing Manager
One Lake Street
Upper Saddle River, New Jersey 07458

The authors may be reached via e-mail at the following addresses:

Dan Limmer   Danlimmer@aol.com
Bob Elling   ellinrob@hvcc.edu

About the Authors

Daniel Limmer is a police officer and paramedic in the Town of Colonie, New York. He is an instructor at the Institute of Prehospital Emergency Medicine at Hudson Valley Community College in Troy, New York. He has been involved in EMS and law enforcement for over 15 years. He is co-author of *Emergency Care, Seventh Edition, First Responder: A Skills Approach, Fourth Edition*, and *Essentials of Emergency Care*.

Bob Elling, MPA, REMT-P is the Program Coordinator for the Hudson Valley Community College Institute of Prehospital Emergency Medicine in Troy, New York. He is also a paramedic with the Town of Colonie, EMS Department. Bob has served as a paramedic for NYC*EMS, Associate Director of the New York State EMS Program, Education Coordinator for Emergency Medical Update, and is the author of the Workbook that accompanies *Emergency Care, Seventh Edition* as well as the co-author of *Essentials of Emergency Care*.

LESSON

1-1 Introduction to EMS Systems

DOT OBJECTIVES

Cognitive Objectives

At the completion of this lesson, the First Responder student will be able to:

1-1.1   Define the components of Emergency Medical Services (EMS) systems.

1-1.2   Differentiate the roles and responsibilities of the First Responder from other out-of-hospital care providers.

1-1.3   Define medical oversight and discuss the First Responder's role in the process.

1-1.4   Discuss the types of medical oversight that may affect the medical care of a First Responder.

1-1.5   State the specific statutes and regulations in your state regarding the EMS system.

Affective Objectives

At the completion of this lesson, the First Responder student will be able to:

1-1.6   Accept and uphold the responsibilities of a First Responder in accordance with the standards of an EMS professional.

1-1.7   Explain the rationale for maintaining a professional appearance when on duty or when responding to calls.

1-1.8 Describe why it is inappropriate to judge a patient based on a cultural, gender, age, or socioeconomic model, and to vary the standard of care rendered as a result of that judgment.

Psychomotor Objectives

No psychomotor objectives identified.

QUICK REVIEW As a First Responder you are a part of an Emergency Medical Services system. The EMS system is activated by dialing "911" in many parts of the country. An "enhanced 911" system allows the emergency medical dispatcher to see a display of the address the person is calling from.

The EMS system includes EMS personnel, as well as Emergency Medical Dispatchers, and hospital personnel such as physicians, nurses, and allied health personnel. Within the EMS system there are four nationally recognized levels of training: First Responder, EMT-Basic, EMT-Intermediate, and Paramedic. The First Responder is trained to respond to emergencies as the first trained person at the scene. The EMT-Basic is designed to be the minimum staffing for an ambulance. EMT-Intermediates and Paramedics perform at advanced levels, trained in invasive skills and to administer medications. With each certification level, the number of training hours and other requirements increase.

As a First Responder, you are trained to arrive at the scene first and render lifesaving care. Your responsibilities include your personal safety as well as the safety of the crew, patient, and bystanders. You are also responsible to make a patient assessment and perform care based on that assessment. You will also need to reassure patients and make them comfortable during the time you spend with them. You will be called upon to assist the EMS units that will continue care of the patients. This will include the efficient transfer of information and assisting with lifting and moving patients. You will need to maintain accurate records of your activities.

The attributes of a First Responder include keeping a neat, clean appearance and a positive image. Patients must be treated with respect and dignity and without regard to race, gender, social status, or any other personal factor. You must keep up to date with your knowledge and skills. This includes patient care skills as well as maintaining knowledge of local, state, and national issues affecting EMS. Develop a good practice ethic and realize that issuance of your certification is simply the beginning of your EMS career.

Medical oversight is a relationship between EMS providers and the physician responsible for out-of-hospital emergency care. The physician responsible for your agency's medical issues is called the *medical director*. There are two types of medical oversight, direct and indirect. *Direct medical oversight* is also referred to as *on-line medical oversight*. In this case, there is actual contact between a physician and a field provider at the scene of an emergency or en route to the hospital. This contact may be via radio, phone, or with an on-scene physician. The on-line physician is not always your medical director. *Indirect medical oversight* does not involve direct contact with a physician. Protocols, quality management, and education are responsibilities of the medical director, indirectly, or "behind the scenes."

When you act as a First Responder you may be acting as a *designated agent* of your medical director. When your medical director issues protocols and you apply these protocols to a patient, you may be acting on an extension of the medical director's authority. This varies from state to state. Always maintain a familiarity with your state and local regulations for all aspects of your duties as a First Responder.

REVIEW QUESTIONS

1. An Emergency Medical Services system is:
   A. the same as an Emergency Medical Technician.
   B. a system that must be staffed with Paramedics.
   C. a network of resources that comes together to provide emergency care to victims of illness or injury.
   D. a centrally located local trauma center that can handle any emergency.

2. The term *First Responder* may include:
   A. firefighter first response.
   B. industrial response teams.
   C. off-duty personnel who come upon a scene.
   D. all of the above.

3. Which of the following is not a direct part of the Emergency Medical Services system?
   A. Emergency Medical Dispatcher
   B. Bystanders

C. EMT-Basic

D. First Responder

4. Which of the following statements about the role of the First Responder is true?
   A. The First Responder is the recommended level of training to staff an ambulance.
   B. The First Responder is the highest level of EMS training.
   C. The First Responder is trained to evaluate the scene and provide lifesaving care until the arrival of the EMT-B.
   D. First Responder certification is only open to firefighters.

5. The First Responder has more training than the EMT-B.
   A. True
   B. False

6. Patient care may vary from person to person due to race, culture, gender, or social status.
   A. True
   B. False

7. Which of the following statements about the role of a First Responder is false?
   A. First Responders have an important role in the EMS system.
   B. First Responders work with EMT-Bs at emergency scenes.
   C. The exact responsibilities of First Responders may vary from region to region.
   D. First Responders are never allowed to deal with medical oversight.

8. A First Responder is responsible for all of the following except:
   A. report writing and record keeping.
   B. gaining access to the patient.
   C. identifying life-threatening conditions.
   D. being able to drive at high speeds in any condition.

9. First Responders are responsible for providing initial patient care based on assessment findings.
   A. True
   B. False

10. Which of the following is the first concern that a First Responder should have upon reaching an emergency scene?
    A. Documenting the mechanism of injury
    B. Airway, breathing, and circulation
    C. Scene safety
    D. Calling for advanced life support (ALS)

11. A First Responder arrives at the scene of a motor vehicle accident. One car is occupied, resting on its side against a utility pole. Which of the following actions would the First Responder do first?
    A. Attempt to perform an immediate rescue, if it could be done quickly.
    B. Pull the first response vehicle in close to check for wires down.
    C. Contact the trauma center and tell them to prepare for patients.
    D. Size up the scene; call for rescue and the power company.

12. The difference between 911 and enhanced 911 (E-911) is:
    A. E-911 is used only by police departments.
    B. E-911 does not display the location of the caller, 911 does.
    C. E-911 displays the location of the caller, 911 does not.
    D. There is no difference between the two systems.

13. Which of the following is not a professional attribute of a First Responder?
    A. Maintains knowledge and skills
    B. Projects a positive image
    C. Maintains knowledge of issues affecting EMS locally and nationally
    D. Placing the safety of the patient before his or her own safety

14. The First Responder may remain on scene after the EMT-Bs arrive and assist with patient care.
    A. True
    B. False

15. Which of the following statements regarding medical oversight is correct?
    A. An example of on-line medical oversight includes standing orders.
    B. Communication with a base station physician must be done over the radio.

C. Medical oversight includes education and quality management.

D. Off-line medical direction is not available to the First Responder.

16. Medical oversight is:
    A. a relationship between the first responder and the physician responsible for out-of-hospital care.
    B. a system where a physician must be on every call.
    C. a physician who is responsible for the quality improvement program only.
    D. none of the above.

17. The term *designated agent* when referring to the relationship between the physician and First Responder means that:
    A. the First Responder designates that physician authority to be medical control on a given call.
    B. the First Responder is acting under the direction, and possibly the license, of the supervising physician.
    C. the physician is employed by the hospital to which the patient will be brought.
    D. none of the above.

18. Your agency's medical director stops at an accident scene and provides direction on patient care. This is an example of on-line medical oversight.
    A. True
    B. False

19. Your local protocols say that you may use your automated external defibrillator (AED) before contacting medical oversight. This ability to use your AED immediately is called a(n):
    A. off-line directive.
    B. on-line directive.
    C. base station physician order.
    D. none of the above.

20. Your local protocols state that after defibrillating a patient three times, you must contact a physician via radio or phone. That contact with the physician and any orders given by the physician are called:
    A. off-line medical direction.
    B. on-line medical direction.

C. indirect medical oversight.

D. none of the above.

1. C. The EMS system is a network of resources that comes together to provide emergency care to victims of illness or injury. All of the other choices represent only one portion of the system. The EMS system begins with the call to the emergency medical dispatcher and includes every contact the patient has through the hospital.

2. D. The First Responder may be any number of people and professions, including all of the choices listed here. When the curriculum was designed, it was meant for the person who arrives first.

3. B. First Responders, EMT-Bs, Advanced EMTs, and Emergency Medical Dispatchers, as well as hospital personnel are considered a part of the EMS system. Bystanders are not a part of the system.

4. C. The purpose of the First Responder level of certification is to provide lifesaving treatment as the first person on the scene. The First Responder will also assist EMT-Bs when possible. The EMT-B is designed to be the minimum level of training for staffing an ambulance.

5. B. The First Responder has fewer hours of training than that for other levels of EMS provider, such as the EMT-B or advanced providers. Remember, the First Responder training program is focused to knowledge and skills that are most important for the first minutes at the scene.

6. B. Patient care must *never* change due to a person's race, gender, culture, or social status. All patients are created equal! The only acceptable means of determining patient treatment is by performing a thorough assessment.

7. D. First Responders, according to the 1995 National Standard Curriculum, are entitled to consult with medical oversight. The other choices are all correct. This question brings out an important point: There will be times when the National Standard Curriculum is not the same as the current practice in your region. The National Registry cannot possibly create an exam that covers what everyone does. They stick to the objectives. When answering test questions on the Registry exam you should, too!

8. D. First Responders must write reports and realize that these reports will be kept as legal records. You will also be responsible for gaining access to the patient and assessing the patient for life-threatening conditions. It is not necessary to drive at high speeds in all conditions. High speeds are dangerous whether you are driving with lights and sirens or not. Always drive safely and you will arrive uninjured to care for your patient.

9. A. First Responders provide initial care based on assessment findings. The initial assessment is perhaps the most important part of patient care and includes airway, breathing, and circulation. It is a major focus of the First Responder's responsibilities.

10. C. Of the choices listed, scene safety is the first concern. If you do not assure your safety, you may be injured and will be of no help to the patient. The other choices are important but are secondary to your safety.

11. D. In this situation, your safety comes first. It would not be safe to drive the vehicle close to the scene or to attempt to remove patients from an unstable vehicle. Calling the trauma center is acceptable to do, but this will not be the first thing you will do. The scene size-up is the first part of any call. Calling for additional resources immediately will allow trained persons to handle the dangers present at the scene.

12. C. Although not available everywhere, 911 is moving closer to being a national emergency phone number. E-911, also called enhanced 911, displays the location the caller is calling from on the emergency dispatcher's screen.

13. D. Safety is always your primary concern. Although television examples or good intentions may cause you to place the safety of others before your own, it is not correct for your safety or for the exam.

14. A. Although the First Responder performs an important role by arriving first, you may still be able to assist EMT-Bs and Advanced Life Support personnel after they arrive. When the EMT-Bs arrive, they are responsible for the patient. Be sure to turn over to the EMT-Bs the information you have learned in your assessment and care.

15. C. Medical oversight is involved in all aspects of emergency care. This includes education and quality management. Off-line medical oversight includes situations where a physician is not contacted directly. On-line oversight involves direct contact with a physician. It may be by radio, telephone, cellular phone, or in person.

16. A. Medical oversight is a relationship between the First Responder and the physician who is ultimately responsible for out-of-hospital care. Oversight may be performed in a number of ways, including protocols, on-line direction, system design, and quality management.

17. B. When you perform patient care in EMS you may be acting under the authority of your agency's medical director. This is referred to as being a designated agent. In some areas you are actually acting under the license of the physician.

18. A. The major distinction between on-line and off-line medical oversight is the direct contact with the physician seen in on-line oversight. The physician on-scene fits the direct contact test and is considered on-line medical oversight.

19. A. Standing orders or protocols are orders that are issued in writing by a physician which allow First Responders and other out-of-hospital providers to perform tasks they would not be allowed to perform without the order. Automated defibrillation is a good example. Since the order is in writing and does not require actual contact with a physician, it is an off-line directive.

20. B. Contacting a physician by radio or phone for any reason is considered on-line medical direction.

1-2

The Well-Being of the First Responder

Cognitive Objectives

At the completion of this lesson, the First Responder student will be able to:

1-2.1 List possible emotional reactions that the First Responder may experience when faced with trauma, illness, death, and dying.

1-2.2 Discuss the possible reactions that a family member may exhibit when confronted with death and dying.

1-2.3 State the steps in the First Responder's approach to the family confronted with death and dying.

1-2.4 State the possible reactions that the family of the First Responder may exhibit.

1-2.5 Recognize the signs and symptoms of critical incident stress.

1-2.6 State possible steps that the First Responder may take to help reduce/alleviate stress.

1-2.7 Explain the need to determine scene safety.

1-2.8 Discuss the importance of body substance isolation (BSI).

1-2.9 Describe the steps the First Responder should take for personal protection from airborne and bloodborne pathogens.

1-2.10 List the personal protective equipment necessary for each of the following situations:
- Hazardous materials
- Rescue operations
- Violent scenes
- Crime scenes
- Electricity
- Water and ice
- Exposure to bloodborne pathogens
- Exposure to airborne pathogens

Affective Objectives

At the completion of this lesson, the First Responder student will be able to:

1-2.11 Explain the importance for serving as an advocate for the use of appropriate protective equipment.

1-2.12 Explain the importance of understanding the response to death and dying and communicating effectively with the patient's family.

1-2.13 Demonstrate a caring attitude towards any patient with illness or injury who requests emergency medical services.

1-2.14 Show compassion when caring for the physical and mental needs of patients.

1-2.15 Participate willingly in the care of all patients.

1-2.16 Communicate with empathy to patients being cared for, as well as with family members and friends of the patient.

Psychomotor Objectives

At the completion of this lesson, the First Responder student will be able to:

1-2.17 Given a scenario with potential infectious exposure, the First Responder will use appropriate personal protective equipment. At the completion of the scenario, the First Responder will properly remove and discard the protective garments.

1-2.18 Given the above scenario, the First Responder will complete disinfection/cleaning and all reporting documentation.

Emotional Aspects of Emergency Care

While some calls are rewarding, others are clearly stressful. Calls such as multiple-casualty incidents, and those involving children, death, violence, and abuse, may evoke a stress response in the First Responder. This stress may be from individual calls or develop over a period of time. The First Responder will also encounter family members and bystanders who are experiencing extreme levels of stress.

First Responder stress has warning signs. These include: irritability, inability to concentrate, anxiety, guilt, and indecisiveness, as well as difficulty sleeping, loss of appetite, loss of interest in sex, feelings of isolation, and loss of interest in work. When these signs and symptoms are noted, actions may be taken to correct them. Lifestyle changes such as changing your diet, avoiding alcohol and fatty foods, exercise, and relaxation may help. If possible, try to change to a less stressful duty assignment or one that allows more time for family and friends.

Stress is often worsened by the reaction of family and friends to your role as a First Responder. It appears that people who are not a part of the EMS system "just don't understand." This leads to a feeling of isolation. Friends and family also fear feeling separated from the First Responder. On-call work with unpredictable schedules add to the stress.

Critical incident stress debriefings (CISDs) are a way of dealing with the stress that results from calls such as multiple-casualty incidents or the death of a child or co-worker. The debriefing is held within 24 to 72 hours of the critical incident. The debriefing is a confidential session where EMS personnel can openly discuss their thoughts and feelings about a call. It is important that the sessions not critique the event. The facilitator of the debriefing offers suggestions on how to deal with the stress. Another type of stress management session is the *defusing*. This session is held a few hours after an event to allow for an initial ventilation of feelings. These may eliminate the need for a formal debriefing or set the groundwork for the full debriefing when it is held. A defusing usually lasts less than an hour. Some experts recommend meditation, visual imagery, and relaxation techniques as additional measures to combat stress.

Dying patients and their families have specific reactions to death and dying. These reactions vary but are generally considered to fall into five categories or stages. Remember, everyone's personal response to stress will vary. The categories are: denial or disbelief ("Not me."), anger ("Why me?"), bargaining ("OK, but first let me . . . "), depression, and finally, acceptance. Remember that anger and other feelings caused by the dying process are sometimes vented on the First Responder. Be tolerant and use good communication skills to help patients and families through this stage of their grieving. Patients and families must be treated with respect. They also need to preserve their dignity, privacy, and a sense of control.

Body Substance Isolation/Scene Safety

Although it is true that there may be risks involved in providing emergency care, most can be fully avoided with attention to certain procedures. This section of the curriculum covers body substance isolation and scene safety.

First Responders may be exposed to infectious diseases when treating patients. The First Responder must assess each call and patient for potential risk and take appropriate action and precautions to eliminate that risk. Actions and equipment for body substance isolation include:

1. Frequent handwashing

2. Proper cleaning, disinfection, and replacement of equipment

3. Gloves, used to prevent contact with blood or body fluids

4. Utility gloves, for cleaning

5. Eye protection, needed to prevent contamination from airborne diseases and splashing substances (goggles are not required)

6. Gowns, used for splashing of fluids as seen in major trauma or childbirth

7. Masks, used to protect the First Responder from blood or fluid spatter reaching the mucous membranes of the mouth and nose

8. OSHA Approved N95 or HEPA (high-efficiency particulate air) respirators, used by EMS providers when patients have suspected tuberculosis

9. Surgical masks, placed over a patient's mouth to prevent transmission of some airborne diseases

Your protection from infectious diseases may also include immunizations against hepatitis B and tetanus. Some agencies require or recommend testing for tuberculosis every six months or yearly as well as testing for immunity against hepatitis B (titer).

Scene safety is an important concept. It entails assuring that the scene is safe from toxic substances, unstable surfaces such as water or ice, violence, or unstable vehicles or conditions at crash scenes. Assuring scene safety is always a first priority. The First Responder may also be responsible for looking out for the safety of the patient and bystanders at an emergency scene. Never enter an unsafe scene! Either take actions which you are trained to perform that will make the scene safe or call for someone who can.

Hazardous materials are common in almost every setting. To identify hazardous substances, the First Responder should carry binoculars so that identification may be made from a distance. Placards are triangular labels placed on vehicles that carry hazardous materials. The book *Hazardous Materials, The Emergency Response Handbook* is a resource for obtaining information about hazardous materials and the appropriate response in an emergency. The bottom line is that "haz-mat" emergencies are to be handled by appropriately trained teams. First Responders only treat patients who have been decontaminated and only after the substance has been contained.

Motor vehicle crashes pose dangers from unstable vehicles, fire, explosion, haz-mat, downed wires, and passing traffic. Jagged metal and glass may also cause injury if appropriate protective equipment is not worn.

Violence may also be faced by the First Responder. It is important to realize that a violent scene must be controlled by law enforcement personnel before the First Responder enters. Observation is critical to prevent entering a scene that is violent or potentially violent. Violent scenes may also be crime scenes. Do not disturb anything unless it is necessary to provide medical care. Your observations are important. Your interaction at a crime scene may require court testimony.

REVIEW QUESTIONS

1. Which of the following may cause a stress response in a First Responder?
   A. Amputations
   B. Elder abuse
   C. Injury of a co-worker
   D. All of the above

2. The stages of death and dying include:
   A. denial, anger, bargaining, depression, and acceptance.
   B. denial, tolerance, depression, and silence.
   C. individual, familial, and community.
   D. denial, dignity, rage, respect, and finally, death.

3. Every patient and family reacts to death and dying in the same manner.
   A. True
   B. False

4. The denial or disbelief stage of death and dying is best characterized by which statement?
   A. "OK, but first let me . . . ."
   B. "Not me."
   C. "Why me?"
   D. none of the above

5. The bargaining stage of death and dying is characterized by which statement?
   A. "OK, but first let me . . . ."
   B. "Not me."
   C. "Why me?"
   D. none of the above

6. Which of the following statements about the acceptance stage of death and dying is most correct?
   A. The patient is happy about dying.
   B. The patient often requires more support than the family.
   C. The family often requires more support than the patient.
   D. In this stage the patient cannot accept the concept of death.

7. Which of the following statements about the needs of the dying patient's family is false?
   A. The family will wish to be treated with dignity.
   B. The family may need to express rage or anger.
   C. The family will need to be controlled.
   D. The family may need to share some of their feelings.

8. Which of the following statements about the actions of the First Responder when dealing with a dying patient or his family is false?
   A. Offer reassurances to give strength, even though they may not be true.

B. Use a reassuring touch if appropriate.

C. Listen.

D. Use a gentle tone of voice.

9. Which of the following are warning signs of stress for the First Responder?

A. Irritability

B. Rapid decision making

C. Increased interest in work

D. All of the above

10. Which of the following actions may be helpful in reducing stress?

A. Increasing caffeine intake

B. Balancing family, work, health, and so on

C. Taking a busier assignment to forget about the stress

D. Alcohol intake

11. Which of the following actions may be helpful in reducing stress?

A. Allowing more time to relax with family and friends

B. Meditation

C. Visual imagery

D. All of the above

12. The nature of the First Responder's activities may cause problems with families and friends. These problems include:

A. increased understanding and tolerance.

B. fear of separation or being ignored.

C. increased ability to communicate.

D. none of the above.

13. Critical incident stress debriefings (CISDs) are usually held within _____ hours of the incident.

A. 2 to 4

B. 12

C. 24 to 72

D. 96 to 120

14. Which of the following statements about critical incident stress is false?

A. The stress is an abnormal reaction to a normal situation.

B. The stress may be caused by a multiple-casualty incident.

C. The stress may be caused by a call involving pediatric trauma.

D. Maintaining an overall state of health and wellness will help combat stress.

15. The difference between a critical incident defusing and a debriefing is:
A. the defusing is usually longer than the debriefing.
B. the defusing is held after the debriefing.
C. the defusing is usually shorter than the debriefing.
D. the debriefing is held immediately after the incident.

16. A critical incident stress team includes:
A. mental health professionals only.
B. mental health professionals and peer counselors.
C. a video recorder for evidence purposes.
D. none of the above.

17. In reference to the risk of infectious disease while treating a patient, the First Responder must:
A. know the infection status of each patient.
B. use all equipment on every call in order to prevent infection.
C. evaluate the potential for exposure and act accordingly.
D. avoid patient contact whenever possible.

18. Handwashing is an essential part of infection control.
A. True
B. False

19. Which of the following statements about the use of protective eyewear is true?
A. Goggles must be worn on every call.
B. Eyewear is not necessary unless you have open wounds around the eye.
C. Personal eyewear may be used if side shields are added.
D. None of the above are true.

20. A multiple-trauma patient has arterial bleeding. Which infection-control items should be worn?
A. Gloves only
B. Gloves and mask only
C. Gloves, mask, and gown only
D. Gloves, mask, gown, and eyewear

21. Which of the following diseases may a First Responder be given a vaccine to develop immunity against?
    A. Acquired immune deficiency syndrome/HIV
    B. Tuberculosis
    C. Meningitis
    D. Hepatitis B (HBV)

22. The First Responder has a responsibility to address the safety of which of the following?
    A. The First Responder himself or herself
    B. The patient
    C. Bystanders
    D. All of the above

23. The First Responder may enter an uncontained hazardous material site *only* to rescue a critical patient.
    A. True
    B. False

24. Which of the following statements about motor vehicle crashes is false?
    A. Vehicles involved in the collision may be unstable.
    B. Downed power lines are considered safe if the power is out to the surrounding areas.
    C. Vehicles at the scene may catch fire or explode.
    D. First Responders face a significant danger from oncoming traffic.

25. Which of the following actions at a crime scene is not the responsibility of the First Responder?
    A. Scene safety
    B. Helping to preserve the scene for evidence
    C. Searching for perpetrators
    D. Treating the victim of the crime

ANSWERS WITH RATIONALE

1. D. All of the call types presented may cause a stress response. The response to stress is an individual reaction and varies from person to person. Other calls that may cause stress include calls which involve children, multiple casualties, and death.

2. A. The stages of death and dying are denial, anger, bargaining, depression, and acceptance. Each person and family experiences the stages differently.

3. B. The stages of death and dying are stages that many people go through. People and families may not go through every stage, spend a short or long time in each, or experience them in a different order. Remember, the purpose for knowing these stages is to be able to deal with dying patients or their families appropriately.

4. B. The denial stage is characterized by a response of "not me." The patient cannot believe that it is happening to him or her.

5. A. In the bargaining stage, the patient tries to postpone death by making an "agreement." In fact, there is no way to make such an agreement. An example might be "OK, but first let me see my daughter graduate from college."

6. C. It is not unusual for the patient and family to be in different stages of dealing with inevitable death. In the acceptance stage, while the patient is certainly not happy about dying, he or she often requires less support than the family requires. Family members often reach the acceptance stage later than the patient.

7. C. The family of a dying patient will require dignity and the need to express their feelings. These feelings may include rage and anger. The family does not need control. In fact, they may need the opposite. Allow patients and family members to assert control when possible.

8. A. Never offer false reassurances to a dying patient or their family. This gives the appearance that the First Responder does not understand the situation and may actually make things worse. Tone of voice, listening, and even a touch are usually appropriate.

9. A. Irritability is the only one of the choices that is a true warning sign of stress for the First Responder. Choices B and C are actually opposites of the actual responses. First Responders often show a decreased interest in work, anxiety, inability to concentrate, indecisiveness, guilt, loss of appetite, and a loss of interest in sex. If you chose D for this question, you may wish to consider reading the question more slowly and carefully.

10. B. A proper balance between work and your health and family is very important. Caffeine and alcohol intake are considered bad for stress. Increasing your workload or hours of work would probably compound the problem.

11. D. All of the choices are actions that would be helpful in reducing stress. Many First Responders don't think of relaxation techniques, meditation, or visual imagery as everyday methods of dealing with stress, but they are!

12. B. Your EMS duties may cause friends and families to feel separated from you or ignored. EMS is an activity that can be very consuming of your time and interest. Be sure to allow time for your family and friends.

13. C. A critical incident stress debriefing (CISD) is usually held within 24 to 72 hours of an incident. A defusing is held within a few hours of the incident.

14. A. Stress is a *normal* response to an *abnormal* situation or circumstance. Choice A states the reverse of this and is thereby false. The other choices are true; multiple-casualty incidents and pediatric trauma may cause stress, and maintaining overall health will help combat stress.

15. C. A defusing is usually shorter than a debriefing. The purpose of a defusing is to allow for initial venting immediately after an incident. A defusing usually lasts only 30 to 45 minutes and may enhance the formal debriefing, which will be held in 24 to 72 hours.

16. B. Although debriefings may vary slightly from area to area, they usually consist of mental health professionals and peer counselors. A debriefing is confidential and is not designed to be a critique, so there would not be a video recorder in the room.

17. C. Since it is not realistic to know the infection status of each patient, and since you cannot avoid patient contact, the correct answer is C. You must understand the concept of infection control and apply it on every call. This would be done by understanding about infectious body substances and appropriate methods to protect yourself from being exposed. Wearing all equipment on every call is not an appropriate solution.

18. A. Handwashing is an essential part of infection control! Many First Responders feel that handwashing is not necessary when gloves are worn. *This is not true!* Wash your hands after all patient contacts and occasionally throughout the day.

19. C. You may use your personal eyeglasses for infection control purposes, but only if you have attached clip-on side protection. Goggles are not necessary if the proper eyeglasses are worn. Eye protection is required any time the potential exists for body substances coming in contact with the eyes. The eyes are surrounded by mucous membranes that could absorb another person's body fluids. This can occur even without open wounds.

20. D. All the items listed must be worn. Gloves will protect the hands, a gown will protect clothing from soiling, and the mask and eyewear protect the mucous membranes of the face (mouth, nose, and eyes).

21. D. Hepatitis B is the only disease for which a vaccination currently exists. A series of three vaccinations over a six-month period will usually provide immunity against the disease. You must still take precautions against infectious diseases, however, because the immunization protects against only one of many diseases.

22. D. While the First Responder's first priority is to protect himself or herself, the First Responder is also charged with looking out for the safety of patients and bystanders.

23. B. This statement is false. All untrained people must stay out of the contaminated areas. Entering this area will cause harm to you and create additional patients. If you enter you will become contaminated and unable to treat the patient you were there to help.

24. B. Downed power lines are always considered to be "live" until they have been moved by the utility company. Assuming that any wire is not charged because of an absence of sparking or power in the area is extremely hazardous. Unstable vehicles, fire, and oncoming traffic are all real hazards.

25. C. The First Responder is primarily responsible for patient care at the crime scene. You should always be conscious of scene safety. Preserving evidence is also important, as long as patient care is not jeopardized. First Responders *should not* participate in hazardous activities such as searching for perpetrators.

1-3 Legal and Ethical Issues

D O T
OBJECTIVES

Cognitive Objectives

At the completion of this lesson, the First Responder student will be able to:

1-3.1 Define the First Responder scope of care.

1-3.2 Discuss the importance of Do Not Resuscitate [DNR] (advance directives) and local or state provisions regarding EMS application.

1-3.3 Define consent and discuss the methods of obtaining consent.

1-3.4 Differentiate between expressed and implied consent.

1-3.5 Explain the role of consent of minors in providing care.

1-3.6 Discuss the implications for the First Responder in patient refusal of transport.

1-3.7 Discuss the issues of abandonment, negligence, and battery and their implications to the First Responder.

1-3.8 State the conditions necessary for the First Responder to have a duty to act.

1-3.9 Explain the importance, necessity and legality of patient confidentiality.

1-3.10 List the actions that a First Responder should take to assist in the preservation of a crime scene.

1-3.11 State the conditions that require a First Responder to notify local law enforcement officials.

1-3.12 Discuss issues concerning the fundamental components of documentation.

Affective Objectives

At the completion of this lesson, the First Responder student will be able to:

1-3.13 Explain the rationale for the needs, benefits and usage of advance directives.

1-3.14 Explain the rationale for the concept of varying degrees of DNR.

Psychomotor Objectives

No psychomotor objectives identified.

QUICK REVIEW *Scope of care* refers to a set of responsibilities that define your conduct and activities as a First Responder. State legislation largely defines your scope of care. An example of this legislation might define which interventions may be performed legally. Your medical director may also issue policies or standing orders that affect your patient care activities. Standing orders are orders issued by the medical director that allow you to perform a certain treatment without having to contact medical oversight. Some systems have a medical oversight system available where physicians may be contacted by phone or radio for consultation on certain issues.

The First Responder also has a series of ethical responsibilities. These include making the physical and emotional needs of the patient a priority, to attend training sessions and maintain proficiency in your skills and knowledge, to strive constantly to improve, and honesty in reporting.

Consent is an important concept for the First Responder. Although it is true that *competent* patients have the right to refuse care, the definition of competent is very important. The failure to provide care, or providing care against a patient's will, can result in legal liability, lawsuits, and possibly arrest. Competence refers to the patient's ability to understand the implications of the decisions they make in reference to their care. Factors that might render a patient incompetent to make these decisions include intoxication or drug use, serious injury, or mental incompetence.

There are several types of consent. Expressed consent may be given by a patient who is competent and of legal age. The patient must be informed about the care they receive and the potential risks. Unconscious patients may be treated under a concept called *implied consent*. This means that the law allows First Responders to treat unconscious patients under the assumption that they would consent to lifesaving care if they were conscious. Children and mentally incompetent adults require the consent of their parent or guardian before care may begin. The definition of "child" and the age of consent vary from state to state. Generally, care may be provided to seriously injured children or incompetent adults in the absence of the parent or guardian based on implied consent. Children that have their own children or those that are emancipated may also be able to give consent.

Patients do have the right to refuse care. In cases of terminal illnesses, a Do Not Resuscitate (DNR) order is a legal document that directs First Responders and other EMS personnel not to resuscitate a patient. Also called advance directives, they usually require the signature of a physician. When there is a question as to whether or not to resuscitate a patient, it is usually better to begin resuscitation.

Any patient may refuse care. This may happen for a number of reasons. Only patients who are competent and of legal age may refuse care. This refusal may occur at any time during your contact with a patient. A patient could regain consciousness and then choose not to go to the hospital. Refusal of care may be a cause for liability for the First Responder. A patient who refuses care must be fully informed and understand the potential risks of refusing care. Generally, First Responders will not be the person making the decision not to transport; others in the EMS system will participate in the process.

Unlawfully touching patients without their consent may result in charges of assault and battery against the First Responder. Negligence is deviation from an accepted standard of care which results in harm to the patient. Several components are necessary to prove a negligence case. The First Responder must have a duty to act. A duty to act may exist simply by being dispatched on a call or by stopping at a roadside accident. The First Responder may breach that duty by failing to act or by acting inappropriately. If injuries occur as a result, the basis exists for a negligence complaint. The injuries may be physical or psychological.

Patients have the right to confidentiality. This includes information obtained in the patient history and assessment, care given, and observations that you make in the privacy of the patient's home. Releasing information may be done only in specific situations. These include information given to others who will care for the patient and judicial subpoena. Your state laws may require mandatory reporting of crimes such as child or elder abuse, domestic violence, rape, and gunshot wounds.

When faced with a crime scene, patient care is a priority. Do not disturb anything unless it is necessary to do so for patient care. Your observations may be important later. Remember that your documentation may be used as evidence in court.

Documentation is important for many reasons. It is vital to transfer information to other health care providers, to document your findings and actions, and to protect you from potential liability. Documentation should be legal, legible, objective, clear, and concise.

Medical identification devices provide important information about a patient's condition. These devices may be found as necklaces, bracelets, or wallet cards. Other programs instruct people to leave information on their medical history and medications in specific places in the house, such as the refrigerator.

REVIEW QUESTIONS

1. Which of the following is not a part of determining a First Responder's scope of care?
   A. State legislation
   B. Medical oversight
   C. Confidentiality
   D. Protocols or standing orders

2. Which of the following is not one of the ethical responsibilities of a First Responder?
   A. Honesty
   B. Maintaining skills and knowledge
   C. Placing the physical and emotional needs of the patient's above your own
   D. Placing the safety of the patient over your own safety

3. Competence, as it applies to patient consent and refusal, is:
   A. the ability to identify the person, place, and date.
   B. the ability to understand implications of decisions affecting care.
   C. any patient who is not intoxicated.
   D. none of the above.

4. Consent is best defined as:
   A. the right to refuse resuscitation for a terminally ill patient.
   B. the acceptance of care by a patient who is informed about his or her care.
   C. obtaining medical oversight's permission to treat the patient.
   D. none of the above.

5. Which of the following patients could not be treated based on the principle of implied consent?
   A. An unconscious adult trauma patient
   B. A competent adult patient with minor injuries
   C. A critically injured child when the parent is not present
   D. A terminally ill patient in cardiac arrest

6. Expressed consent requires all of the following except:
   A. informing the patient of care you will give and any risks involved.
   B. the patient must be competent and of legal age.
   C. the patient must be less than 18 years of age.
   D. none of the above.

7. You respond to a call for a "person down." You arrive to find an unconscious patient with an obvious head wound. You may begin care based on which principle:
   A. expressed consent
   B. consent of incompetent adults
   C. law enforcement consent
   D. implied consent

8. You respond to the residence of a patient in cardiac arrest. Family members meet you at the door and advise you that the patient has a terminal illness and does not want to be resuscitated. They have no forms or legal paperwork. You should:
   A. begin resuscitation of the patient.
   B. honor the family's wishes and do nothing.

C. call the patient's physician before deciding on a course of action.

D. do nothing and wait for the EMT-Bs.

9. Competent adults have the right to refuse medical care and/or transportation.
   A. True
   B. False

10. Assault and battery charges may result from:
    A. informing the patient of risks involved with treatment.
    B. touching or transporting patients against their will.
    C. failure to act.
    D. breach of duty.

11. Turning the patient over to EMT-Bs at the scene and leaving may result in charges of abandonment.
    A. True
    B. False

12. Which of the following is not a component of negligence?
    A. Duty to act
    B. Injury and/or damages were inflicted
    C. Criminal intent
    D. The actions of the First Responder caused the injury or damage

13. A patient may file a lawsuit for negligence if psychological damages alone occur.
    A. True
    B. False

14. Once the dispatcher tells a caller that help is on the way, a duty to act exists.
    A. True
    B. False

15. Which of the following does not constitute a breach of duty?
    A. Failing to act
    B. Acting appropriately
    C. Acting inappropriately
    D. None of the above

16. Which of the following statements about confidentiality is false?
    A. Generally, small amounts of information may be given out over the phone.
    B. Release of information requires written permission from the patient.
    C. It is acceptable to provide necessary information to other health care providers who will be treating this patient.
    D. Some mandatory reporting situations (child abuse, etc.) do not require a signed release.

17. After scene safety has been addressed, the first priority of the First Responder at a violent crime scene is the preservation of evidence.
    A. True
    B. False

18. Which of the following statements about a First Responder's actions at a crime scene is false?
    A. Do not disturb things unnecessarily.
    B. Your call report could be used in court as evidence.
    C. Your observations of the scene are important.
    D. First Responders cannot be called into court to testify due to medical immunity.

19. Medical identification devices may be observed as:
    A. bracelets.
    B. necklaces.
    C. wallet cards.
    D. all of the above.

20. First Responder call reports may be used in court as evidence.
    A. True
    B. False

ANSWERS WITH RATIONALE

1. C. Your scope of practice as a First Responder is the group of laws and regulations that define what you may do. This may include state legislation, medical oversight, protocols, and standing orders. Confidentiality is another legal principle that does not have anything to do with scope of practice.

2. D. You should never place the safety of the patient over your own safety. If you become injured, you will not be able to help your patient. Becoming a patient yourself will add another patient and be a burden on the EMS system. Honesty, maintaining your skills, and watching out for the physical and emotional needs of patients are all responsibilities of a First Responder.

3. B. Competence is the ability to understand implications of decisions affecting care. If patients are to make any decisions regarding their care, they must understand the pros and cons of that decision. Understanding person, place, and date is orientation, not competence. Lack of intoxication may be a part of competence, but not the entire concept.

4. B. Consent must be informed; that is, the patient must understand the care that he or she is about to receive. The patient must know the potential risks and benefits of this care. Consent does not involve permission from medical oversight. In most cases, even a physician cannot force care on competent patients against their will.

5. B. A competent adult patient with minor injuries may not be treated based on implied consent. Being competent, the patient may make their own decisions. All of the other patients here could be treated based on implied consent. The principle of implied consent is based on the fact that a reasonable person would consent to care if he or she were conscious. Even in the case of a pediatric or terminally ill patient, implied consent may be used.

6. C. To give consent, a patient must be competent and of legal age. Choice C states that the patient must be *less than* 18 years of age. This goes against the need to be of legal age to provide consent. Every exam you take will have questions that require careful reading and concentration. This is one of those questions.

7. D. Since the patient is unconscious, implied consent allows you to treat the patient. Remember, implied consent means that it is assumed (or implied) that the patient would consent to care if he or she were conscious. The law allows you to believe that the patient still wants your care. Expressed consent can only be given by conscious, competent patients. Consent of incompetent adults and law enforcement consent have no bearing here.

8. A. As a First Responder you will come upon calls such as this one. The correct answer is to begin resuscitation of the patient. A Do Not Resuscitate (DNR) order would allow you not to begin resuscitation. If you waited for someone to call the doctor, then found that the doctor wanted resuscitation begun, you have wasted valuable

minutes. Although the family may be correct about the terminal illness, begin care unless there is a legal reason not to. Always follow your local protocols.

9. A. Competent patients do have the right to refuse care and transportation. The patient must be advised of the potential risks of doing so. The patient may also be required to sign a release or waiver to protect you from liability.

10. B. Patients generally have the right to refuse care. Bodily forcing care or transportation upon a patient could result in criminal or civil charges of assault and/or battery.

11. B. Turning patients over to someone with *less* training than you have is abandonment. This is not the case here. Since the patient was turned over to an EMT-B, which is a higher level of care than First Responder, it is not considered abandonment.

12. C. Criminal intent is not required to prove a case of negligence. Negligence requires a duty to act, a breach of that duty, and injuries or damages caused because of the actions of the First Responder.

13. A. In a negligence case, the damages do not have to be physical. Psychological or emotional damages are sufficient grounds for a lawsuit.

14. A. A duty to act does exist once the dispatcher tells a caller that help is on the way. If you stop at an accident scene while on duty, you have also created a duty to act. The definition of a duty to act becomes less clear when you are off-duty or out of your response area. Following your conscience and providing care will almost always be right.

15. B. Acting appropriately is not a breach of duty. Failing to act when required, or acting inappropriately, constitutes a breach of duty.

16. A. Giving information out over the phone, even in small amounts, without a release is wrong. Even with a release, you may not be able to identify the caller and release information to the wrong person. Release of information requires the patient's signature giving permission. Exceptions are information given about a patient's condition to another person caring for the patient and some mandatory reporting situations.

17. B. The first priority at a crime scene, after scene safety is addressed is taking care of the patient. Although you should always

try to preserve evidence, do so only if it can be done without jeopardizing your patient.

18. D. First Responders are often called into court as witnesses in criminal trials because they arrive first, sometimes even before the police. The other choices are all correct statements about First Responders and crime scenes.

19. D. Medical identification devices come in many forms, including bracelets, necklaces, and wallet cards. Some communities have programs where medical information is stored in a vial inside the refrigerator or in another specific location.

20. A. The reports you prepare as a First Responder are legal documents and may be called into court as evidence. The documents must be completed neatly and accurately.

1-4 | The Human Body

DOT OBJECTIVES

Cognitive Objectives

At the completion of this lesson, the First Responder student will be able to:

1-4.1 Describe the anatomy and function of the respiratory system.

1-4.2 Describe the anatomy and function of the circulatory system.

1-4.3 Describe the anatomy and function of the musculoskeletal system.

1-4.4 Describe the components and function of the nervous system.

Affective Objectives

No affective objectives identified.

Psychomotor Objectives

No psychomotor objectives identified.

QUICK REVIEW

Knowledge of the anatomy, or structure, of the human body is important information for a First Responder. This knowledge will help you to identify injured areas and communicate effectively with other EMS providers. Your understanding of anatomy and the way that body systems function will be an essential foundation of knowledge that will help you in your studies and patient care situations.

Musculoskeletal System

The musculoskeletal system gives the body shape, protects many of the body's vital organs, and enables the body to move. This system consists of muscles, bones, and the tissues that connect muscles and bones to each other.

The *skeletal system* consists of bones and includes the following:

1. The skull, which houses and protects the brain

2. The spinal column, which houses and protects the spinal cord

3. The bones of the torso:
   a. The ribs, which encircle the chest and meet the sternum (breastbone).
   b. The xiphoid process, the lowest portion of the sternum, which is used to locate hand position for CPR compressions.

4. The pelvis, a series of bones that form the hips

5. The lower extremities, formed by a series of bones:
   a. The femur (thigh), the largest long bone in the body.
   b. The patella (knee cap).
   c. The tibia and fibula, bones of the lower leg (shin).
   d. The bones of the ankle, feet, and toes.

6. The bones of the upper extremity:
   a. The bones of the shoulder: clavicle (collar bone) and scapula (shoulder blade).
   b. The humerus (upper arm).
   c. The radius and ulna (lower arm).
   d. The bones of the wrist, hand, and fingers.

Joints are where bones connect to other bones. Examples of joints are knees, elbows, and shoulder joints.

Muscles are another important component of the musculoskeletal system. There are three types of muscles: voluntary, involuntary, and cardiac.

1. *Voluntary muscles*, also known as *skeletal muscles*, are attached to bones and are responsible for movement. They can be contracted or relaxed under the conscious control of the body.

2. *Involuntary muscles*, also known as *smooth muscles*, are found in the digestive and urinary tracts as well as in the blood vessels and respiratory system. These muscles, as their name implies, are not under our conscious control.

3. *Cardiac muscle*, found only in the heart, comprises specialized involuntary muscles and are responsible for circulating blood throughout the body. Cardiac muscle is very sensitive to reduced levels of oxygen.

Respiratory System

The respiratory system is responsible for bringing oxygen into the body and for removal of carbon dioxide from the body. This is done through a process called *respiration*. When inhalation occurs, the diaphragm moves down and the chest moves out, causing air to be drawn into the lungs. For exhalation, the opposite happens. The diaphragm rises and the chest moves inward, causing air to exit the lungs.

The components of the respiratory system are as follows:

1. The nose and mouth.

2. The oropharynx, the area at the rear (posterior) of the mouth, but above the vocal cords.

3. The nasopharynx, the open area posterior to the nose.

4. The epiglottis, a leaf-shaped structure that protects the trachea from foreign objects.

5. The trachea, or windpipe, a structure formed by cartilage rings that carries air into the lungs.

6. The larynx, or voice box, where vocal cords are located.

7. The two lungs.

8. The diaphragm, a muscular organ that assists in breathing by contracting and lowering which causes air to flow into the lungs. Relaxation results in the diaphragm rising and air being forced from the lungs.

9. The bronchi, tubes that gradually decrease in size. They carry air from the trachea to the alveoli.

10. The alveoli, small structures in which air and carbon dioxide are exchanged with the blood.

There are differences between the airways of adults and those of infants and children. Some of these differences include:

1. The airway structures of infants and children are smaller and more easily obstructed.

2. Infants' and children's tongues take up proportionately more space in the mouth than do adults'.

3. The trachea of an infant or child is more flexible than that of an adult.

4. Infants and children do not usually have cardiac problems. Cardiac arrest in infants and children is caused by a problem with *respiration*, making airway control and ventilation very important.

Circulatory System

The circulatory system takes oxygen from the respiratory system and delivers it to tissues throughout the body. Nutrients are also transported throughout the body. The circulatory system removes waste products from the tissues and transports these products to be removed from the body.

The primary component of the circulatory system is the *heart*, a four-chambered organ. The two upper chambers are called *atria*, the two lower chambers are called *ventricles*. Blood returning from the body enters the right atrium and is pumped into the right ventricle. The blood leaves the right ventricle and travels to the lungs, where it picks up oxygen. Oxygenated blood returns to the left atrium, then the left ventricle, and finally out of the heart through the aorta to the body. The heart has valves between its chambers to prevent blood from flowing backward.

When the left ventricle of the heart contracts, blood is pumped into circulation. This contraction of the left ventricle is done at high pressure and creates the "pulse" that is felt throughout the body where arteries pass close to bones.

Arteries carry blood away from the heart and are under high pressure. *Veins* carry blood back to the heart. *Capillaries* are the smallest type of blood vessel and are where nutrients and waste products are exchanged with the cells of the body. Important arteries to know are:

- *Carotid*, the major artery of the neck. This is the artery that is checked when assessing for a pulse during CPR.

- *Femoral*, located in the thigh. This artery may be palpated near the crease between the groin and the upper thigh.

- *Radial*, located at the thumb side of the wrist. It is used commonly for obtaining a pulse in a conscious patient.

- *Brachial*, an artery in the upper arm. It is used commonly as a pressure point to control bleeding to the arm.

Nervous System

The nervous system controls voluntary and involuntary activity in the body. It also allows us to think, feel, and display emotion. The nervous system may be divided into two subsystems:

1. *Central nervous system:* the portion of the nervous system that contains the brain and spinal cord.

2. *Peripheral nervous system:* the portion of the nervous system responsible for sensation and movement throughout the body. It is broken down into two types of response:
   a. *Sensation:* carries information from the body to the spinal cord and to the brain.
   b. *Motor:* carries information from the brain through the spinal cord and to the body.

The Skin

The skin, although not thought of as an organ, or even as being very important, actually serves major functions. These functions include:

1. Protecting the body from the environment and dangerous organisms such as bacteria.

2. Participation in temperature regulation of the body and in prevention of dehydration.

3. Sensing heat, cold, pressure, pain, and transmitting these stimuli to the brain through peripheral nerves.

REVIEW QUESTIONS

1. Which of the following is not a function of the musculoskeletal system?
   A. Provides shape
   B. Protects vital organs
   C. Produces nervous system impulses
   D. Provides movement

2. Which of the following organs or structures are not a part of the musculoskeletal system?
   A. The skull (cranium)
   B. The brain
   C. The humerus (upper arm)
   D. The femur (thigh)

3. The lowest portion of the sternum is called the:
   A. xiphoid process.
   B. mandible.
   C. thorax.
   D. manubrium.

4. Voluntary muscle would be found in the
   A. heart.
   B. lungs.
   C. legs.
   D. intestines.

5. Involuntary muscle may be found in all of the following except the:
   A. urinary system.
   B. blood vessels.
   C. bronchi.
   D. finger.

6. Which of the following statements correctly describes the events during inhalation?
   A. The diaphragm moves downward and the ribs move out.
   B. The diaphragm moves upward and the ribs move out.
   C. The diaphragm moves downward and the ribs move in.
   D. The diaphragm moves upward and the ribs move in.

7. The leaf-shaped structure that folds down and prevents foreign material from entering the trachea is called the:
   A. windpipe.
   B. bronchi.
   C. larynx.
   D. epiglottis.

8. The diaphragm is located:
   A. between the lungs.
   B. beneath the lungs and above the abdomen.

C. around the trachea.

D. above the trachea to prevent foreign material from entering.

9. The alveoli are:
   A. small, grapelike clusters within the lungs where gas exchange takes place with the blood.
   B. small, grapelike clusters throughout the body where gas exchange takes place with the cells.
   C. cartilage rings around the trachea.
   D. special cells found only in the heart that allow electrical conduction.

10. Which of the following statements regarding the airways of infants and children is true?
    A. Airway structures are proportionately larger in children than in adults.
    B. The trachea is more flexible in children than in adults.
    C. The tongues of children are proportionately smaller in children than in adults.
    D. All of the above are true statements.

11. The primary cause(s) of cardiac arrest in children is/are:
    A. poisoning.
    B. heart deformities.
    C. uncorrected respiratory problems.
    D. allergic reactions.

12. After leaving the lungs, blood returns to the:
    A. right atrium.
    B. right ventricle.
    C. left atrium.
    D. left ventricle.

13. When returning to the heart from the body, blood goes to the:
    A. right atrium.
    B. right ventricle.
    C. left atrium.
    D. left ventricle.

14. Veins carry blood:
    A. back to the heart.
    B. away from the heart.
    C. through the lungs only.
    D. in the thorax only.

15. The artery in the neck that is used for pulse checks is called the:
    A. brachial.
    B. femoral.
    C. jugular.
    D. carotid.

16. The femoral pulse is located in the area of the:
    A. neck.
    B. upper arm.
    C. groin.
    D. wrist.

17. A pulse may be felt in the body due to the contraction of the:
    A. right atrium.
    B. right ventricle.
    C. left atrium.
    D. left ventricle.

18. The radial pulse is located in the:
    A. neck.
    B. upper arm.
    C. groin.
    D. wrist.

19. The central nervous system consists of the:
    A. heart, lungs, arteries, and veins.
    B. brain and spinal cord.
    C. nerves in the arms and the legs.
    D. cranium (skull) and spinal column.

20. Peripheral nerves are responsible for:
    A. sensation and motor response.
    B. respiratory control.
    C. cardiac control.
    D. thought processes, consciousness, and emotion.

ANSWERS WITH RATIONALE

1. C. The musculoskeletal system provides shape, protects vital organs, and provides movement. It does not produce or originate nervous system impulses.

2. B. The skull (cranium), the humerus, and the femur are all bones, or parts of the body comprised of bones and are therefore part

of the musculoskeletal system. The brain is an organ and is part of the central nervous system. It is not part of the musculoskeletal system.

3. A. The lowest part of the sternum is called the xiphoid process. You may have heard of this area during CPR training. The xiphoid is used as a landmark to locate proper hand compressions during CPR. If you have not taken your CPR training yet, you will hear about the xiphoid again soon.

4. C. Voluntary muscles would be found in the legs. The legs are under conscious control and are voluntary. Conscious control means that you can move a body part when you want. The other choices here are not in the same category. The heart, lungs, and intestines are involuntary and will work without you thinking about them.

5. D. Similar to the preceding question, involuntary muscles are present in the urinary system, blood vessels, and bronchi. They are not present in the finger.

6. A. During inhalation the diaphragm moves downward and the ribs move out. This provides for expansion of the chest cavity and the inward flow of air.

7. D. The epiglottis is the leaf-shaped structure that folds down over the trachea to prevent foreign material from entering. The "windpipe" is the trachea itself, the bronchi are smaller tubes that branch off the trachea, and the larynx is the "voice box" or area that contains the vocal cords.

8. B. The diaphragm is located below the lungs and above the abdominal cavity. In fact, it is the diaphragm that separates the abdominal cavity from the chest cavity or thorax. The diaphragm is very important in breathing.

9. A. The alveoli are grapelike clusters that are within the lungs. They are the smallest unit of the lung, where air exchange takes place with the blood. Alveoli are located only within the lungs.

10. B. The trachea of an infant or child is more flexible than that of an adult. This means that they could be injured more easily. The other choices are false. Airway structures in children are proportionately smaller in children and the tongues of children are proportionately larger.

11. C. The primary causes of cardiac arrest in children are respiratory problems. The majority of children do not have heart

attacks or other problems that adults face, but respiratory problems that prevent breathing or reduce oxygen intake do cause death in infants and children. This is why so much emphasis is placed on airway care for infants and children.

12. C. After leaving the lungs, blood returns to the left atrium. The left side of the heart receives blood from the lungs. The left ventricle, the most muscular chamber of the heart, receives blood from the left atrium and pumps the oxygenated blood to the entire body.

13. A. The right atrium receives blood that is returning to the heart from the body. The blood is no longer oxygenated and carries waste products. The right atrium pumps the blood to the right ventricle, then to the lungs to pick up oxygen and leave waste products.

14. A. Veins carry blood back to the heart. Arteries carry blood away from the heart.

15. D. The artery in the neck that is used for pulse checks is the carotid. The brachial pulse is in the upper arm, the femoral near the groin. The jugular vein is also located in the neck but is a vein and cannot be used for pulse checks.

16. C. As noted in the rationale above, the femoral pulse is located in the area of the groin. The pulse in the wrist is called the radial pulse.

17. D. A pulse is felt in the body, due to the contraction of the left ventricle. This is a strong muscular chamber that contracts, sending blood throughout the body.

18. D. The radial pulse is located in the wrist. It is located on the lateral aspect, the side closer to the thumb.

19. B. The central nervous system consists of the brain and spinal cord. The nerves in the arms and legs are part of the peripheral nervous system. The cranium and spinal column are the bony structures that protect the central nervous system, not the system itself.

20. A. Peripheral nerves are responsible for sensation and motor response. The other choices are those that are functions of the central nervous system.

1-5 Lifting and Moving Patients

DOT
OBJECTIVES

Cognitive Objectives

At the completion of this lesson, the First Responder student will be able to:

1-5.1 Define body mechanics.

1-5.2 Discuss the guidelines and safety precautions that need to be followed when lifting a patient.

1-5.3 Describe the indications for an emergency move.

1-5.4 Describe the indications for assisting in non-emergency moves.

1-5.5 Discuss the various devices associated with moving a patient in the out-of-hospital arena.

Affective Objectives

At the completion of this lesson, the First Responder student will be able to:

1-5.6 Explain the rationale for properly lifting and moving patients.

1-5.7 Explain the rationale for an emergency move.

Psychomotor Objectives

At the completion of this lesson, the First Responder student will be able to:

1-5.8 Demonstrate an emergency move.

1-5.9 Demonstrate a non-emergency move.

1-5.10 Demonstrate the use of equipment utilized to move patients in the out-of-hospital arena.

QUICK REVIEW The term *body mechanics* refers to the way we use our bodies to lift and move patients. Lifting and moving must be performed properly to prevent injury to the patient and First Responder. Proper patient transportation may improve a patient's condition or at least prevent that condition from deteriorating. Lifting and moving patients causes many injuries to First Responders each year; some injuries are so serious they end a career. There are guidelines that must be followed while lifting and moving patients. These include using your legs, not your back, to lift; and keeping the weight you are lifting as close to your body as possible.

You should position your feet squarely on the ground when lifting and never twist during the lifting process. Evaluate the weight of the patient and the need for extra help. The terrain the patient must be moved over is another important consideration. Be aware of your physical abilities and limitations. When working with others, be sure to communicate clearly and frequently during the lifting process.

In general, patient moves fall into two categories: emergency and nonemergency (nonurgent) moves. An *emergency move* is performed when there is an immediate danger to the patient if he or she is not moved quickly. Examples of situations where an emergency move would be used include fire or danger from explosion, inability to protect the patient from dangers at the scene, or the inability to access another patient in a vehicle who requires lifesaving care. Another example of an emergency move would be when a patient could not be given emergency care because of the patient's position or location (i.e., moving a patient to a flat, solid surface to perform CPR).

With emergency moves comes the risk of worsening an existing spinal injury. Since the life-threatening problem requires you to move the patient, use a long-axis drag to minimize the movement of the spine. The long-axis drag usually involves dragging the patient from the head and shoulders so that the spine will stay in a relatively straight line. Dragging sideways, such as by an arm will cause the spine to move in a way that can cause serious injury. Other moves and drags, such as the clothing drag or blanket drag, may be used.

When none of the conditions mentioned above exist, *nonemergency moves* should be used. These are usually done by the EMS crew after the patient has been assessed, treated, and is ready for transportation. There are a wide variety of nonemergency moves. These include the direct ground lift, where two or three rescuers lift the patient directly off the ground; the extremity lift, where the patient is lifted by two rescuers, one at the shoulders and the other at the knees; and the draw sheet method, where the patient is moved by lifting or sliding a sheet that is under the patient. These nonemergent moves are only for patients who do not have spinal injury (or the potential for spinal injury). Refer to your textbook to obtain detailed information on moves and carries.

As a First Responder, your actions in deciding whether the patient must be moved and how to do it are very important. It is also important to know how to position a patient without causing further injury until the EMS crew arrives. Patients with trauma should not be moved until their injuries can be stabilized. The obvious exception is the patient who requires airway care, CPR, or is in a life-threatening situation.

Unresponsive patients without spine injury are placed in the recovery position. In this position the patient is placed on his or her side (often the left side) with the arm closest to the ground outstretched and supporting the head and a knee bent to keep the patient in position. This allows for drainage of the mouth and helps to prevent airway problems. Patients experiencing pain or respiratory distress are placed in a position of comfort. Often this is a sitting position. The patients must be monitored carefully for airway status and vomiting. A position of comfort should not be used for spine-injured patients.

Your first response unit may carry transportation devices or you may be called to assist EMS units that do. Ambulances have a wheeled stretcher or cot that is used to transport the patient to and from the ambulance and to carry the patient while in the ambulance. There are a variety of portable devices used in EMS. The *orthopedic* or *scoop stretcher* splits in half lengthwise. The two halves are placed alongside the patient and brought together to scoop the patient onto the device. The scoop stretcher is useful for lifting but does not provide spinal immobilization. The *stair chair* is a wheeled device that transports a patient in the sitting position. As its name implies, the device is ideal for use on stairs and when the patient is uncomfortable lying flat. There are portable stretchers made of various materials that may be used at multiple-casualty incidents or for difficult moves.

There are various types, styles, and brands of backboards or *spineboards*. These are generally broken down into long spineboards, which immobilize the entire body, and short spineboards, which secure the head, neck, and torso. There are specialty brands of short boards, such as the KED®, Kansas®, and LSP Halfback® spineboards. Read and follow the manufacturer's recommendations for each device.

REVIEW QUESTIONS

1. Body mechanics is best defined as:
   A. work done by an orthopedic surgeon.
   B. the way we use our bodies to lift and move patients.
   C. the procedure for performing an emergency move.
   D. the position to place an unresponsive patient for least resistance.

2. Which of the following is not part of the First Responder's duties in lifting and moving?
   A. Moving patients who are in immediate danger
   B. Assisting other EMS personnel to lift and move patients
   C. Positioning patients to prevent further injury
   D. Moving patients who are not in danger prior to EMT's arrival

3. Which of the following statements regarding safe lifting is true?
   A. Lift with your legs, not your back.
   B. Lift with your back, not your legs.
   C. Keep the weight as far away from your body as possible.
   D. Do not twist while lifting unless your feet are positioned properly.

4. Which of the following are guidelines for safe lifting?
   A. Make sure that your feet are positioned properly.
   B. Determine whether help is necessary prior to lifting.
   C. Communicate with your partner prior to lifting.
   D. All of the above are guidelines for safe lifting.

5. Emergency moves are:
   A. moves that are done in nonemergent situations.
   B. moves that are performed when there is an immediate danger to the patient.
   C. moves that may only be performed when the victim is in cardiac arrest.
   D. moves that require an EMT-B or above to perform.

6. The major concern when performing an emergency move is that:
   A. spine injuries may be aggravated or worsened.
   B. applying a short spineboard takes a long time.
   C. completing the full detailed exam must be done first.
   D. there are no hazards associated with the move.

7. Nonemergent moves are performed:
   A. with only one First Responder.
   B. when patients require immediate life-threatening care.
   C. with EMT-Bs and other responders when hazards are not present.
   D. only after radio contact with medical direction.

8. When referring to patient movement, the term *long axis* means the:
   A. patient must be moved on a spineboard.
   B. patient is dragged by an arm or leg to prevent spine compression.
   C. move may only be performed on tall patients.
   D. move is performed so that the patient's spine is kept in line.

9. Which of the following is not an indication for an emergency move?
   A. A vehicle containing occupants is on fire.
   B. A patient inside a vehicle requires extrication.
   C. A patient must be moved because she cannot protect her own airway.
   D. You must reach another patient who requires lifesaving care.

Answer questions 10 to 12 based on the following scenario.
You arrive at a motor vehicle accident to find that a car has run into a tree. You have access only to the passenger side of the vehicle. Passenger A in the front passenger seat has head and neck pain but

appears conscious and alert. Patient B, who is in the driver's seat, is unconscious and appears to have a considerable amount of blood in his mouth. His respirations are noisy.

10. Passenger A would require which type of patient movement?
    A. Emergency move
    B. Nonemergency move
    C. No movement until the EMT-Bs arrived
    D. None of the above

11. Passenger B would require which type of patient movement?
    A. Emergency move
    B. Nonemergency move
    C. No movement until the EMT-Bs arrived
    D. None of the above

12. If either patient A or B were moved on emergency basis, the main complication that you would suspect from this move would be:
    A. injuries sustained from applying the short spineboard.
    B. possible airway problems from waiting for the EMT-Bs.
    C. spine injuries or complications from the urgent nature of the move.
    D. none of the above are possible.

13. Which of the following is not an emergency move?
    A. Long-axis drag
    B. Clothing drag
    C. Kendrick Extrication Device (KED) application
    D. Blanket drag

Answer questions 14 to 16 based on the following scenario.
You are a First Responder who is called to a car that was struck in the rear by another vehicle. The collision accident occurred at relatively low speeds. The driver of the vehicle that was struck complains of pain in his neck. He is conscious and alert without further complaints. There are no hazards noted.

14. The patient in this scenario would receive which type of movement from the First Responders upon their arrival at the scene?
    A. Emergency move
    B. Nonemergency move

C. No movement until the EMT-Bs arrived

D. None of the above

15. If the patient in the scenario also complained of back pain, he would receive which type of move?

A. Emergency move

B. Nonemergency move

C. No movement until the EMT-Bs arrived

D. None of the above

16. If the engine compartment of the vehicle in the scenario was on fire, which move would you perform on the patient?

A. Emergency move

B. Nonemergency move

C. No movement until the EMT-Bs arrived

D. None of the above

17. Generally, nonemergency moves are performed after the EMT-Bs arrive at the scene and treat the patient.

A. True

B. False

18. A conscious patient experiencing respiratory difficulty or chest pain who does not have spinal injury is usually placed:

A. in the recovery position.

B. in a left laterally recumbent position.

C. on a long spineboard.

D. in a position of comfort.

19. The recovery position is used primarily for:

A. unconscious patients without trauma.

B. conscious patients with pain.

C. traumatic injuries to the head or neck.

D. none of the above.

20. Which of the following transportation devices is acceptable to use in a spine-injured patient?

A. Stair chair

B. Portable stretcher

C. Long spineboard

D. Canvas stretcher

1. B. Body mechanics is best defined as the way we use our bodies to lift and move patients. Lifting and moving patients is an important part of your responsibilities as a First Responder. It is also important for preventing injury to yourself during the lifting process.

2. D. First Responders are responsible for lifting and moving patients who are in danger, or those whose conditions require movement prior to arrival of the EMT-Bs. Patients who are not in danger or those who do not require movement because of their condition (airway problems, etc.) would not be moved before the EMT-Bs arrive.

3. A. Answer A is true. You must always lift with your legs, not your back. Choice B states the opposite of choice "a." Choice "c" is incorrect. You must keep the weight you are lifting as close to your body as possible. Choice "d" is incorrect because you should avoid twisting while lifting, regardless of the position of your feet.

4. D. All of the choices listed are correct. You should always position your feet properly, determine whether help is necessary before lifting, and communicate with your partner.

5. B. Emergency moves are those that are performed when there is an immediate danger to the patient. Examples include the risk of fire or explosion. They may also be performed when the patient requires immediate care (such as CPR), or when the patient must be moved to access another patient who requires lifesaving care.

6. A. The major concern with emergency moves are that spine injuries may be worsened. It is an accepted risk, however, because if you chose an emergency move, the alternative would be death or significant additional injury caused by the dangers present and not moving the patient. The other choices do not apply. Short spineboards are not used in emergency moves of adults, so the time it takes to apply one is not a consideration. Detailed examinations are not usually completed first, so this answer is also incorrect. The final choice is not correct since there are hazards associated with an emergency move, but the hazards of moving the patient are less than those of leaving the patient in danger.

7. C. The First Responder National Standard Curriculum states that nonemergency moves should not be performed by First Responders. If there is no reason for an emergent move, the correct answer is to wait for the EMT-Bs. You may find that your EMS system has provided additional training and allows you to perform nonemergency moves prior to the EMT-B's arrival. If this is the case,

your local examination may vary from the National Registry examination. Ask your course instructor for details.

8. D. In a long-axis move the patient's spine is kept close to its natural shape and position. An example of an in-line move is the shoulder drag. Most moves that keep in-line spinal position are done from the head and shoulder area. Although spineboards are ideal, they are not always practical for emergency moves. Dragging by the arm or leg will cause the spine to bend, which will clearly worsen preexisting injury. The height of the patient is not a factor in long-axis moves.

9. B. Choice B is not an indication for an emergency move. It simply states that the patient requires extrication without providing information on hazards or patient condition. The other choices—fire, airway problems, and reaching another person who requires lifesaving care—are all clear indications for an emergency move.

Questions 10 to 12 are based on a scenario preceding the questions. When reading this or any scenario, make sure that you read carefully. One missed bit of information about the scene could make all your choices incorrect. In this scenario the critical information to look at is the position of the vehicle and the condition of the patients.

10. A. This is a difficult question. It bases the answer on your knowledge of moves *and* your analysis of the scenario. Although patient A does not have injuries that would require an emergency move, access is limited to passenger B because the car is against a tree on the passenger side. Passenger A requires an emergency move because passenger B requires lifesaving care due to an airway problem.

11. A. This is more clear cut. Passenger B is unconscious and has "considerable blood" in his mouth, which poses an immediate threat to his airway.

12. C. As stated in an earlier question, the primary complication of emergency moves is the risk of worsening an existing spinal injury. This paints a clear picture of when emergency moves are used: when the risk of spinal injury is outweighed by the potential of death from a hazard or uncorrected problems (airway, bleeding, etc.).

13. C. A KED (Kendrick Extrication Device) application is not an emergency move because in an emergency move, a spinal immobilization device is not applied. The time it would take to apply the device would be harmful to a patient with airway problems and

dangerous to both the patient and First Responder if a hazard existed. Even though an extrication device was not used, the emergency move may still be done cautiously, and with the speed required to help the patient's condition. The other choices are all recognized emergency moves.

Questions 14 to 16 are based on a scenario preceding the questions. Remember to read carefully!

14. C. This patient does not appear to have life-threatening conditions and there is no indication of danger to the patient. In this case, the First Responder would stabilize the patient's spine and wait for the EMT-Bs to perform spinal immobilization.

15. C. Even though back pain was added to this scenario, without immediate danger or the presence of life-threatening conditions, nothing would change. For this patient, patient movement would be initiated by the EMT-Bs. In most cases, the First Responder will stay and help the EMT-Bs with the spinal immobilization and movement of the patient.

16. A. This alteration to the scenario makes it a clear situation where an emergency move is required. Fire or risk of explosion requires an emergency move, as do life-threatening conditions.

17. A. Nonemergency moves are performed after the arrival of the EMT-B. This is because nonemergency moves are done after a full patient assessment and may require specialized equipment. Remember, this procedure may vary from system to system. What is on the National Registry examination may not be the actual practice in your local EMS system.

18. D. The position of comfort is the position that is recommended for patients who are experiencing respiratory difficulty or chest pain. This "position" may actually be a variety of positions. The most common position is a sitting or semisitting position. It is dependent of what makes the patient comfortable. This position may not be used on patients who have spinal injuries. Patients who are not able to maintain their own airway must not be placed in this position. Monitor patients frequently. If a patient loses consciousness or is unable to maintain his or her own airway, the patient must be moved to an appropriate position.

19. A. The recovery position is used on unconscious patients who do not have spinal injury. The term *recovery position* comes from the fact that this position was initially recommended for patients

who had regained pulse and respirations after CPR. The position was also found to be useful for patients who were unconscious or otherwise unable to protect their airway because it allowed for drainage. The position must not be used for spine-injured patients.

20. C. The only device listed in the choices for this question that is appropriate for a spine-injured patient is the long spineboard. The stair chair transports in a sitting position, which is inappropriate for spine-injured patients. Portable and canvas stretchers do not offer adequate support and immobilization of the spine.

LESSON | **2-1** | **Airway**

D O T
OBJECTIVES **Cognitive Objectives**

At the completion of this lesson, the First Responder student will be able to:

2-1.1 Name and label the major structures of the respiratory system on a diagram.

2-1.2 List the signs of inadequate breathing.

2-1.3 Describe the steps in the head-tilt chin-lift.

2-1.4 Relate mechanism of injury to opening the airway.

2-1.5 Describe the steps in the jaw thrust.

2-1.6 State the importance of having a suction unit ready for immediate use when providing emergency medical care.

2-1.7 Describe the techniques of suctioning.

2-1.8 Describe how to ventilate a patient with a resuscitation mask or barrier device.

2-1.9 Describe how ventilating an infant or child is different from an adult.

2-1.10 List the steps in providing mouth-to-mouth and mouth-to-stoma ventilation.

2-1.11 Describe how to measure and insert an oropharyngeal (oral) airway.

2-1.12 Describe how to measure and insert a nasopharyngeal (nasal) airway.

2-1.13 Describe how to clear a foreign body airway obstruction in a responsive adult.

2-1.14 Describe how to clear a foreign body airway obstruction in a responsive child with complete obstruction or partial airway obstruction and poor air exchange.

2-1.15 Describe how to clear a foreign body airway obstruction in a responsive infant with complete obstruction or partial airway obstruction and poor air exchange.

2-1.16 Describe how to clear a foreign body airway obstruction in a unresponsive adult.

2-1.17 Describe how to clear a foreign body airway obstruction in a unresponsive child.

2-1.18 Describe how to clear a foreign body airway obstruction in a unresponsive infant.

Affective Objectives

At the completion of this lesson, the First Responder student will be able to:

2-1.19 Explain why basic life support ventilation and airway protective skills take priority over most other basic life support skills.

2-1.20 Demonstrate a caring attitude towards patients with airway problems who request emergency medical services.

2-1.21 Place the interests of the patient with airway problems as the foremost consideration when making any and all patient care decisions.

2-1.22 Communicate with empathy to patients with airway problems, as well as with family members and friends of the patient.

Psychomotor Objectives

At the completion of this lesson, the First Responder student will be able to:

2-1.23 Demonstrate the steps in the head-tilt chin-lift.

2-1.24 Demonstrate the steps in the jaw thrust.

2-1.25 Demonstrate the techniques of suctioning.

2-1.26 Demonstrate the steps in mouth-to-mouth ventilation with body substance isolation (barrier shields).

2-1.27 Demonstrate how to use a resuscitation mask to ventilate a patient.

2-1.28 Demonstrate how to ventilate a patient with a stoma.

2-1.29 Demonstrate how to measure and insert an oropharyngeal (oral) airway.

2-1.30 Demonstrate how to measure and insert a nasopharyngeal (nasal) airway.

2-1.31 Demonstrate how to ventilate infant and child patients.

2-1.32 Demonstrate how to clear a foreign body airway obstruction in a responsive adult.

2-1.33 Demonstrate how to clear a foreign body airway obstruction in a responsive child.

2-1.34 Demonstrate how to clear a foreign body airway obstruction in a responsive infant.

2-1.35 Demonstrate how to clear a foreign body airway obstruction in an unresponsive adult.

2-1.36 Demonstrate how to clear a foreign body airway obstruction in an unresponsive child.

2-1.37 Demonstrate how to clear a foreign body airway obstruction in an unresponsive infant.

QUICK REVIEW The First Responder should be able to name and label the *ten major structures of the respiratory system* on a diagram. The following are the structures with their descriptions:

1. Nose: a structure that purifies the air we breathe by catching impurities and warming the air.

2. Mouth: the large opening to the airway and respiratory system which allows the taking in of air and contains the tongue and teeth.

3. Pharynx: an area at the back of the mouth.

4. Oropharynx: inside the mouth posterior to the tongue, leading to the throat.

5. Nasopharynx: the area between the nasal passages and the oropharynx.

6. Epiglottis: a leaf-shaped structure that prevents food and liquid from entering the trachea during swallowing.

7. Windpipe (trachea): the passageway in the front (anterior) of the throat through which air passes during breathing.

8. Voice box (larynx): a structure within the neck in which the vocal cords and glottic opening into the trachea are located.

9. Lungs: the two organs of the respiratory system, which fill with air during inspiration and empty during expiration.

10. Diaphragm: the large primary muscle of breathing which separates the chest (thorax) from the abdomen. Upon inhalation it moves down, and during exhalation it moves back up.

Adequate breathing consists of a normal rate of 12 to 20 breaths per minute in an adult, 15 to 30 for a child, and 25 to 50 for an infant. A patient with adequate breathing should exhibit breath sounds that are equal and present on both sides. The patient should also have visible and symmetric chest expansion with minimal effort. The signs of *inadequate breathing* include:

- A respiratory rate of less than 8 per minute in adults, less than 10 per minute in children, or less than 20 per minute in infants.

- Inadequate chest wall motion, such as unequal from side to side or absent on one side of the chest.

- The patient's skin, lips, tongue, earlobes, or nailbeds are blue (cyanotic) or gray.

- Changes in the patient's mental status.

- Increased respiratory effort.

- Gasping for air or grunting between breaths.

- A slow heart rate associated with slow respirations.

The procedure for opening the airway is dependent on the potential for neck injury. If you are able to rule out any potential trauma to the neck by your observations or those of bystanders, the head-tilt chin-lift should be used. The procedure for the *head-tilt chin-lift* is as follows:

1. Once the patient is in the supine position, place one hand on the forehead and place the fingertips of the other hand under the bony area at the center of the patient's jaw.

2. Use your fingertips to lift the chin and to support the lower jaw. Move the jaw forward to a point where the lower teeth are almost touching the upper teeth.

3. If a patient has no gag reflex, use an oral airway to keep the tongue from occluding his or her airway. In some situations it may be helpful to use the thumb of the hand supporting the chin to pull back the patient's lower lip. To avoid being bitten, do not insert your thumb into the patient's mouth.

If the mechanism of injury leads you to suspect a possible injury to the neck, the standard procedure for airway opening using the head-tilt chin-lift should not be used; rather, the jaw thrust maneuver must be used to open the airway. The procedure for the *jaw thrust* is as follows:

1. Keep the patient's head, neck, and spine aligned, moving him as a unit as you place him in the supine (flat on his back) position. It normally takes more than one First Responder to move the patient into this position, but it can be done carefully with only one. The person holding the neck should direct all movement of the patient.

2. Kneel at the top of the patient's head, resting your elbows on the surface on which the patient is lying.

3. Carefully reach forward and place one hand on each side of the patient's lower jaw, at the angle of the jaw below the ears.

4. Stabilize the patient's head with your forearms while using your index fingers to "jut the jaw" by pushing the patient's lower jaw forward. It is essential that you have your fingers behind the angle of the jaw, not just on the bottom; otherwise, you will just shut the patient's mouth. You may need to retract the patient's lower lip with your thumb to keep the mouth open. Do not tilt or rotate the patient's head since any movement may cause an injury to the cervical spine.

It is important to have a suction unit ready for immediate use when providing emergency medical care. This is because the patient may have secretions, blood, or food particles in the airway which partially occlude the airway or could be aspirated into the lungs. Worse yet, the patient could vomit (an active process) or regurgitate (a passive process), causing the potential for volatile and poisonous substances from the stomach to be aspirated or inhaled into the lungs of the patient. Since the lung tissue is very fragile, aspirated material causes severe pneumonia, which may be fatal.

The principles of *suctioning* involve using negative pressure to keep the airway clear. Use these steps for suctioning:

1. Be sure to observe body substance isolation, as the material you are removing is considered a biohazard.

2. Position yourself at the patient's head and turn the patient to the side if he or she is not at risk of a cervical injury.

3. Measure the catheter. It is not necessary to measure a rigid-tip catheter as long as your do not lose sight of the tip. Use the preferred "tonsil sucker" or rigid tonsil tip (Yankauer) rather than a soft catheter, which is designed to pass down a tube. If using a flexible catheter, measure the same way that you measure for an oropharyngeal airway (OPA).

4. Open the mouth using the cross-finger technique.

5. Place the Yankauer so that the convex (bulging-out) side is against the roof of the patient's mouth. Insert the tip to the base of the tongue. Follow the pharyngeal curvature. Do not push the tip down into the throat or into the larynx.

6. Apply suction only after the Yankauer or catheter tip is in place. Apply suction on the way out, moving the tip from side to side. Limit suctioning to 15 seconds in an adult because you are also removing oxygen from the patient's respiratory system. When suctioning an infant, limit your time to 5 seconds, and with children limit it to 10 seconds.

The procedure for *ventilating* a patient with a resuscitation mask or barrier device is as follows:

1. Take body substance isolation precautions. Wear gloves and an eyeshield. You will be unable to wear a disposable mask.

2. Position yourself at the patient's head and open the airway. If available, insert an OPA to help keep the patient's airway open.

3. Connect oxygen to the inlet on the face mask. Run oxygen at 15 liters or more per minute. Barrier devices such as face shields are usually not designed to be attached to supplemental oxygen.

4. Position the mask on the patient's face so that the apex (pointed end) is over the bridge of the nose and the base is between the lower lip and prominence of the chin.

5. Hold the mask firmly in place while maintaining the proper head tilt. To lift the jaw forward, place both thumbs on the sides of the mask. The index, third, and fourth fingers are placed on each side of the patient's face between the angle of the jaw and the ear lobe. Jut the jaw up to the mask; avoid squeezing the mask down onto the face since this squeezing closes the mouth and airway.

6. Take a deep breath and exhale into the mask's one-way valve at the top of the mask port. Each ventilation should be delivered over 1 1/2 to 2 seconds and contain approximately 800 to 1200 cc in the average adult and 1 to 1 1/2 seconds in infants and children. Watch closely for the patient's chest to rise. Do not overinflate or ventilate too fast, as this will fill the stomach with air and increase the chance of regurgitation.

7. Remove your mouth from the port and allow for passive exhalation. Continue the procedure for ventilating following the rescue breathing and CPR guidelines.

The ventilation rate for adults should be 10 to 12 breaths per minute with a 1 1/2- to 2-second ventilation time. Children and infants should be ventilated at 20 per minute with a 1- to 1 1/2-second inspiratory time. The rate for newborns is 40 per minute with a 1- to 1 1/2-second inspiratory time.

When it becomes necessary to ventilate an infant or child it is essential that you be well practiced in the use of the pediatric-sized pocket mask and a bag valve mask using the correct-size device (either an infant/newborn or child size). Follow these guidelines when ventilating the infant or child patient:

1. Avoid breathing too hard through the pocket face mask or using excessive bag pressure and volume. Use only enough to make the patient's chest rise.

2. Use properly sized face masks to assure a good mask seal.

3. Do not use flow-restricted, oxygen-powered ventilation devices since they are contraindicated in infants and children.

4. If ventilation is not successful in raising the patient's chest, perform the procedures for clearing an obstructed airway, then try to ventilate again.

5. The AHA standards do not allow the use of a "pediatric pop-off valve" on any size BVM.

It is important to know how to use airway adjuncts and avoid mouth-to-mouth contact. However, in some circumstances it may become necessary for the First Responder to provide mouth-to-mouth and mouth-to-stoma ventilation. You should always try to have a barrier device available. Devices must be carried where you work or volunteer. Consider having a device in your car as well as on your key chain. A stoma is a permanent surgical opening in the front of the throat (trachea) for a patient with a laryngectomy to breathe through. The procedure for ventilation is as follows:

1. Wear gloves to take body substance isolation. If a barrier device is available, be sure to use one.

2. Position yourself at the side of the patient's head and do a head-tilt chin-lift on a patient who has not sustained trauma.

3. Look for chest rise and use your ear to listen or feel air exchange from the open mouth.

4. If there is no breathing, cover the entire mouth or stoma with yours and squeeze the nose closed. If the patient has a complete laryngectomy it will not be necessary to seal off the mouth or nose.

5. Ventilate the patient. Each ventilation should be delivered over 1 1/2 to 2 seconds in adults and 1 to 1 1/2 seconds in infants and children. Watch closely for the patient's chest to rise.

6. Remove your mouth and allow for passive exhalation. Continue the procedure for ventilating following the rescue breathing or CPR guidelines.

The First Responder needs to know how to insert both OPA and nasopharyngeal airways (NPAs). The procedure for measuring the oropharyngeal airway is to select a size that fits from the center of the mouth to the angle of the jaw or from the earlobe to the corner of the mouth. The procedure for *OPA insertion* is to:

1. Take body substance isolation precautions.

2. Place the patient on his or her back and open the airway using either the head-tilt chin-lift or jaw thrust maneuver if you suspect trauma.

3. Open the patient's jaw using the cross-fingered technique. Cross the thumb and forefinger of one hand and place them on the patient's upper and lower teeth at the corner of the mouth. Then spread your fingers apart.

4. Position the correct-size airway so that its tip is pointing toward the roof of the patient's mouth.

5. Insert the airway by sliding it along the roof of the patient's mouth, past the soft tissue hanging down from the back (the uvula), or until you meet resistance against the soft palate. Be certain not to push the patient's tongue back into the throat.

6. Now flip the airway 180 degrees over the tongue so that the tip is pointing down into the patient's throat. This prevents pushing the tongue back.

7. Once the OPA has been inserted, place the nontrauma patient in a maximum head-tilt position (hyperextension). Check to see that the airway flange is against the patient's lips. If the airway is too long or short, replace it with the one of proper size.

NPAs are measured by one of the following two methods. Use an NPA that is the diameter of the patient's smallest finger or use one that extends from the tip of the patient's nose to their earlobe. The procedure for *NPA insertion* is to:

1. Take body substance isolation precautions.

2. Lubricate the NPA with a water-based lubricant such as KY jelly, Lubifax, or Surgilube. Do not use an oil-based lubricant

such as Vaseline, which can damage the tissue lining the nasal cavity and if aspirated, can cause pneumonia.

3. Gently push the tip of the nose upward while keeping the patient's head in a neutral position. Most NPAs are designed to be placed in the right nostril. The beveled or angled portion at the tip of the airway should face toward the nasal septum, the wall that separates the nostrils.

4. Insert the airway into the nostril, advancing until the flange rests firmly against the patient's nostril. Never force an NPA. If you experience any difficulty advancing the airway, pull it out, rotate 180 degrees, and try to insert it in the other nostril.

The First Responder must be able to recognize and clear *foreign-body airway obstructions* in responsive or unresponsive patients. The airway can either be clear, partially obstructed, or completely obstructed (blocked). Partial airway obstruction with good air exchange is generally treated by encouraging the patient to cough to clear the airway. Always stand-by during this period, as the obstruction could suddenly become a complete obstruction or poor air exchange could develop. Partial airway obstruction with poor air exchange is treated the same as complete airway obstruction.

The steps in the management of an *unconscious infant* with a foreign-body airway obstruction are as follows:

1. Establish unresponsiveness. If a second First Responder is available, have him or her activate the EMS system.

2. Open the airway and try to ventilate; if still obstructed, reposition the head and try to ventilate again.

3. Give up to five back blows and five chest thrusts.

4. Perform a tongue-jaw lift, and if you see the object, perform a finger sweep to remove it.

5. Repeat steps 2 through 4 until effective. If the patient is breathing or resumes effective breathing, place in the recovery position.

6. If airway obstruction is not relieved after about 1 minute, activate the EMS system.

The steps in the management of a *conscious infant* with a foreign-body airway obstruction are as follows:

1. Confirm complete airway obstruction. Check for serious breathing difficulty, ineffective cough, or no strong cry.

2. Give up to five back blows and five chest thrusts.

3. Repeat step 2 until effective or the patient becomes unconscious.

The steps in the management of an *unconscious child* with a foreign-body airway obstruction are as follows:

1. Establish unresponsiveness. If a second First Responder is available, have him/her activate the EMS system.

2. Open airway and try to ventilate; if still obstructed, reposition head and try to ventilate again.

3. Give up to five abdominal thrusts.

4. Perform a tongue-jaw lift, and if you see the object, perform a finger sweep to remove it.

5. Repeat steps 2 through 4 until effective. If patient is breathing or resumes effective breathing, place in recovery position.

6. If airway obstruction is not relieved after about 1 minute, activate the EMS system.

The steps in the management of a *conscious child* with a foreign-body airway obstruction are as follows:

1. Ask "Are you choking?"

2. Give abdominal thrusts.

3. Repeat thrusts until effective or patient becomes unconscious.

The steps in the management of an *unconscious adult* with a foreign-body airway obstruction are as follows:

1. Establish unresponsiveness. Activate the EMS system.

2. Open airway and try to ventilate; if still obstructed, reposition head and try to ventilate again.

3. Give up to five abdominal thrusts.

4. Perform a tongue-jaw lift followed by a finger sweep to remove the object.

5. Repeat steps 2 through 4 until effective. If patient is breathing or resumes effective breathing, place in recovery position.

The steps in the management of a *conscious adult* with a foreign-body airway obstruction are as follows:

1. Ask "Are you choking?"

2. Give abdominal thrusts (chest thrusts for pregnant or obese patients).

3. Repeat thrusts until effective or patient becomes unconscious.

REVIEW QUESTIONS

1. The leaf-shaped structure that prevents food and liquid from entering the trachea during swallowing is called the:
   A. larynx.
   B. pharynx.
   C. epiglottis.
   D. diaphragm.

2. The structure within the neck in which the vocal cords and glottic opening into the trachea are located is called the:
   A. larynx.
   B. epiglottis.
   C. pharynx.
   D. nasopharynx.

3. Signs of inadequate breathing include:
   A. skin, lips, tongue, or nailbed cyanosis.
   B. increased respiratory effort.
   C. gasping for air or grunting between breaths.
   D. all of the above.

4. Inadequate breathing can be due to a respiratory rate:
   A. of less than 18 per minute in adults.
   B. of less than 20 per minute in infants.
   C. of greater than 8 per minute in children.
   D. none of the above.

5. The procedure for a head-tilt chin-lift includes:
   A. placing one hand on the forehead.
   B. jutting the jaw forward with two hands.

C. kneeling at the top of the patient's head.

D. all of the above.

6. If a patient is found unconscious at the bottom of a stairwell, the First Responder should open the airway using the:

A. jaw thrust.

B. head-tilt chin-lift.

C. head-tilt neck-lift.

D. any of the above.

7. The jaw thrust maneuver is best done:

A. with the patient supine.

B. by kneeling at the top of the patient's head.

C. by jutting the jaw.

D. all of the above.

8. Suction units work best on:

A. thick and granular material.

B. teeth and clots.

C. fluids and blood.

D. all of the above.

9. When suctioning a patient the First Responder should be sure to:

A. suction on the way in.

B. suction on the way out of the mouth.

C. limit your time to 30 seconds.

D. all of the above.

10. When using a rigid tip, the First Responder should:

A. not need to measure the catheter.

B. measure from the nose to earlobe.

C. measure from the center of the mouth to the jaw.

D. none of the above.

11. When resuscitating a patient with a mask:

A. position yourself at the patient's head.

B. open the airway.

C. hold the mask in place while maintaining head tilt.

D. all of the above.

12. Each ventilation on an adult should be:

A. 1/2 to 1 second.

B. 1 to 1 1/2 seconds.

C. 1 1/2 to 2 seconds.

D. 2 to 2 1/2 seconds.

13. The rate of ventilations for adults should be:

    A. 6 to 8 per minute.

    B. 10 to 12 per minute.

    C. 14 to 16 per minute.

    D. 18 to 20 per minute.

14. Children and infants should be ventilated at a rate of:

    A. 5 per minute.

    B. 10 per minute.

    C. 20 per minute.

    D. 40 per minute.

15. Ventilating a child is different from ventilating an adult in that:

    A. the ventilation rate is faster.

    B. flow-restricted oxygen-powered ventilation devices are not used.

    C. the ventilations are smaller in volume.

    D. all of the above.

16. When providing mouth-to-stoma ventilation on an adult be sure to:

    A. remove your mouth to allow passive exhalation.

    B. deliver ventilations over 1 to 1 1/2 seconds.

    C. wear gloves and a mask.

    D. none of the above.

17. A properly sized OPA should extend from:

    A. the angle of the jaw to the corner of the mouth.

    B. the corner of the mouth to the tip of the nose.

    C. the center of the mouth to the angle of the jaw.

    D. all of the above are correct.

18. A properly sized NPA should extend from:

    A. the angle of the jaw to the corner of the mouth.

    B. the tip of the patient's nose to the earlobe.

    C. the corner of the mouth to the nose.

    D. none of the above.

19. When assessing a possible FBAO patient who is a conscious adult:
    A. quickly check the pulse first.
    B. call the ambulance prior to any assessment.
    C. administer five sets of back blows.
    D. ask them if they can speak or are choking.

20. When a patient has a partial airway blockage with poor air exchange, the First Responder should:
    A. provide supplemental oxygen.
    B. treat it like a complete airway blockage.
    C. wait for the patient to pass out.
    D. all of the above.

21. When treating a child with a foreign-body airway obstruction, the First Responder should not:
    A. begin with an abdominal thrust.
    B. automatically do finger sweeps.
    C. use the jaw thrust maneuver.
    D. place the patient in a supine position.

22. The procedure for foreign-body airway obstruction in an unresponsive adult includes:
    A. chest thrusts.
    B. aggressive back blows.
    C. providing abdominal thrust and finger sweeps.
    D. all of the above.

23. When treating a responsive child with a suspected foreign-body airway obstruction, the first responder should first:
    A. determine if there is poor air exchange.
    B. immediately administer back blows.
    C. immediately administer abdominal thrusts.
    D. all of the above.

24. When treating a responsive infant with a complete foreign-body airway obstruction, the first responder should:
    A. start CPR.
    B. administer abdominal thrusts.
    C. provide chest thrusts instead of abdominal thrusts.
    D. reach in and sweep the throat.

25. The indications for chest thrusts include:
    A. pregnant patients.
    B. obese patients.
    C. infants.
    D. all of the above.

1. C. The leaf-shaped structure that prevents food and liquid from entering the trachea during swallowing is called the epiglottis. The larynx is the voice box, the pharynx is the back of the mouth, and the diaphragm is the major muscle of breathing.

2. A. The structure within the neck in which the vocal cords and glottic opening into the trachea are located is called the larynx. The epiglottis is defined in question 1, the pharynx is the back of the mouth, and the nasopharynx is the area between the nostrils and the pharynx.

3. D. Signs of inadequate breathing include: skin, lips, tongue, or nailbed cyanosis, increased respiratory effort, and gasping for air or grunting between breaths.

4. B. Inadequate breathing can be due to a respiratory rate of less than 20 per minute in infants. In adults this is less than 8 per minute, and in children it is less than 10 per minute.

5. A. The procedure for a head-tilt chin-lift includes placing one hand on the forehead. Jutting the jaw forward with two hands is done in the jaw thrust. Kneeling at the top of the patient's head is done when using the jaw thrust and not the head-tilt chin-lift.

6. A. If a patient is found unconscious at the bottom of a stairwell, the First Responder should open the airway using the jaw thrust. The head-tilt chin-lift is used on patients who have no potential trauma. The head-tilt neck-lift is no longer used.

7. D. The jaw thrust maneuver is best done with the patient supine, by kneeling at the top of the patient's head, and by jutting the jaw.

8. C. Suction units work best on fluids and blood. Larger material and granulated material must be scooped out with a gloved finger.

9. B. When suctioning a patient the First Responder should be sure to suction on the way out of the mouth. This will help you limit the amount of oxygen that is being removed from the respiratory system as you are preparing to suction the patient.

10. A. When using a rigid tip the First Responder should not need to measure the catheter. A flexible catheter is measured from the center of the mouth to the angle of the jaw in the same way that an oral airway is sized. The rigid tip is not measured; rather, you just do not lose sight of the tip while suctioning.

11. D. When resuscitating a patient with a mask: position yourself at the patient's head, open the airway, and hold the mask in place while maintaining head tilt.

12. C. Each ventilation on an adult should be 1 1/2 to 2 seconds.

13. B. The rate of ventilations for adults should be 10 to 12 per minute.

14. C. Children and infants should be ventilated at a rate of 20 per minute or once every 3 seconds.

15. D. Ventilating a child is different from ventilating an adult in that: the ventilation rate is faster, flow-restricted oxygen-powered ventilation devices are not used, and the ventilations are smaller in volume.

16. A. When providing mouth-to-stoma ventilation on an adult, be sure to remove your mouth to allow passive exhalation. The ventilations should be given over 2 to 2 1/2 seconds, and it is not possible to wear a mask and blow into a stoma at the same time.

17. C. A properly sized OPA should extend from the center of the mouth to the angle of the jaw. If it extends from the angle of the jaw to the corner of the mouth or from the corner of the mouth to the tip of the nose, it would not be the proper length.

18. B. A properly sized NPA should extend from the tip of the patient's nose to the earlobe. If it was sized from the angle of the jaw to the corner of the mouth or the corner of the mouth to the nose it would not be the proper length.

19. D. When assessing a possible FBAO patient who is a conscious adult, ask them if they can speak or are choking. The patient's response (or lack of a response) will determine which type of obstruction is present.

20. B. When a patient has a partial airway blockage with poor air exchange, the First Responder should treat it like a complete airway blockage. This is because poor air exchange is often as bad as little-to-no air exchange and needs to be corrected immediately. Supplemental oxygen is useful but not essential until the blockage is corrected.

21. B. When treating a child with a foreign-body airway obstruction, the First Responder should not automatically do finger sweeps. You should not put your fingers in the mouth of an infant or child unless you actually see an object that you could grab with your finger tips.

22. C. The procedure for foreign-body airway obstruction, in an unresponsive adult includes providing abdominal thrust and finger sweeps. Back blows are not used on adults, and chest thrusts are used only on obese adults and pregnant patients.

23. A. When treating a responsive child with a suspected foreign-body airway obstruction, the First Responder should determine if there is poor air exchange. Back blows are only done on infants, and abdominal thrusts should not be used until you confirm there is an obstruction.

24. C. When treating a responsive infant with a complete foreign-body airway obstruction, the First Responder should provide chest thrusts instead of abdominal thrusts. Abdominal thrusts are not used on infants, and you should not reach in and sweep the throat of an infant unless you actually see an object that you could grab with your fingertips.

25. D. The indications for chest thrusts include: pregnant patients, obese patients, and infants.

LESSON | **3-1** | Patient Assessment

DOT OBJECTIVES

Cognitive Objectives

At the completion of this lesson, the First Responder student will be able to:

3-1.1 Discuss the components of scene size-up.

3-1.2 Describe common hazards found at the scene of a trauma and a medical patient.

3-1.3 Determine if the scene is safe to enter.

3-1.4 Discuss common mechanisms of injury/nature of illness.

3-1.5 Discuss the reason for identifying the total number of patients at the scene.

3-1.6 Explain the reason for identifying the need for additional help or assistance.

3-1.7 Summarize the reasons for forming a general impression of the patient.

3-1.8 Discuss methods of assessing mental status.

3-1.9 Differentiate between assessing mental status in the adult, child, and infant patient.

3-1.10 Describe methods used for assessing if a patient is breathing.

3-1.11 Differentiate between a patient with adequate and inadequate breathing.

3-1.12 Describe the methods used to assess circulation.

3-1.13 Differentiate between obtaining a pulse in an adult, child, and infant patient.

3-1.14 Discuss the need for assessing the patient for external bleeding.

3-1.15 Explain the reason for prioritizing a patient for care and transport.

3-1.16 Discuss the components of the physical exam.

3-1.17 State the areas of the body that are evaluated during the physical exam.

3-1.18 Explain what additional questioning may be asked during the physical exam.

3-1.19 Explain the components of the SAMPLE history.

3-1.20 Discuss the components of the on-going assessment.

3-1.21 Describe the information included in the First Responder "hand-off" report.

Affective Objectives

At the completion of this lesson, the First Responder student will be able to:

3-1.22 Explain the rationale for crew members to evaluate scene safety prior to entering.

3-1.23 Serve as a model for others by explaining how patient situations affect your evaluation of the mechanism of injury or illness.

3-1.24 Explain the importance of forming a general impression of the patient.

3-1.25 Explain the value of an initial assessment.

3-1.26 Explain the value of questioning the patient and family.

3-1.27 Explain the value of the physical exam.

3-1.28 Explain the value of an on-going assessment.

3-1.29 Explain the rationale for the feelings that these patients might be experiencing.

3-1.30 Demonstrate a caring attitude when performing patient assessments.

3-1.31 Place the interests of the patient as the foremost consideration when making any and all patient care decisions during patient assessment.

3-1.32 Communicate with empathy during patient assessment to patients as well as with family members and friends of the patient.

Psychomotor Objectives

At the completion of this lesson, the First Responder student will be able to:

3-1.33 Demonstrate the ability to differentiate various scenarios and identify potential hazards.

3-1.34 Demonstrate the techniques for assessing mental status.

3-1.35 Demonstrate the techniques for assessing the airway.

3-1.36 Demonstrate the techniques for assessing if the patient is breathing.

3-1.37 Demonstrate the techniques for assessing if the patient has a pulse.

3-1.38 Demonstrate the techniques for assessing the patient for external bleeding.

3-1.39 Demonstrate the techniques for assessing the patient's skin color, temperature, condition, and capillary refill (infants and children only).

3-1.40 Demonstrate questioning a patient to obtain a SAMPLE history.

3-1.41 Demonstrate the skills involved in performing the physical exam.

3-1.42 Demonstrate the ongoing assessment.

Patient assessment is one of the most important skills that a First Responder can possess. If you are to perform lifesaving care, you must be able to detect life-threatening problems. You will find that most patients do not have life-threatening problems. Patient assessment is important for these patients, too. A properly performed patient assessment contains many parts, the most important of which is assuring your own safety. The parts of the patient assessment process are the scene size-up, initial assessment, First Responder physical exam, patient history, and the ongoing assessment.

The *scene sizeup* is the first part of the patient assessment process. The steps of the scene size-up are:

1. *Body substance isolation* (BSI). This must be considered on every call. Body substance isolation precautions consist of gloves, eye protection, gown, and mask. Each should be used when appropriate. It is during the scene size-up that you would evaluate the type of call to anticipate which BSI precautions you would take.

2. *Scene safety*. The main question in this part of the size-up is answering the question: Is the scene safe? The scene may be unsafe from hazardous materials, unstable vehicles or surfaces (slope, ice), or violent situations. Your first priority is to protect yourself. Never enter a hazardous scene. You also have an obligation to protect your patient and even bystanders when possible.

3. *Mechanism of injury* (MOI) or *nature of illness determination*. Since you are examining the scene for dangers you should also observe for a mechanism of injury. This means that you will examine a scene for indications of how the patient was injured and the physical forces involved. Examples include damage to the steering wheel or windshield of a vehicle caused by the patient's body striking these parts during the crash. MOI is used in trauma patients. Nature of illness is the equivalent for medical patients. Here you will determine from the patient, family or bystanders why EMS was called.

4. *Resource determination*. This is the final section of the size-up. Before beginning care, determine if any other resources are needed to handle the scene safely and efficiently. This step includes determining the number of patients, and calling for additional ambulances and EMS providers, utility companies, the fire department, law enforcement, or specialized teams. It is important to call for help *before* beginning care. You will be

less likely to remember to call for help once you begin providing care. *Triage* is a system of sorting patients by treatment priority. This system is used in cases where there are multiple patients. Multiple-casualty incidents (MCIs) and triage are discussed in Chapter 14.

The *initial assessment* begins the hands-on patient care portion of the assessment. The purpose of the initial assessment is to identify and treat immediate threats to life. The steps of the initial assessment are:

1. *General impression.* This is determined from your immediate assessment of the environment and the patient's chief complaint. You need to determine whether the patient is a medical or trauma patient. Some patients may be both while others are difficult to determine. If in doubt, treat the patient as a trauma patient to prevent additional spinal injury. You will also determine the patient's gender and approximate age. Developing a general impression will also be an early indicator of the patient's condition so appropriate actions may be taken.

2. *Determine responsiveness.* Begin by speaking to the patient. Remember to stabilize the spine as soon as you suspect potential spine injury. Tell the patient your name, that you are a trained First Responder, and that you are there to help. Patients may be in any level of consciousness. A scale to use for level of consciousness is *AVPU* which stands for *a*lert, *v*erbal, *p*ain, or *u*nresponsive. If the patient does not respond verbally, you may need to apply a safe but painful stimulus to test the patient's response. The patient who does not respond to a properly applied painful stimulus is truly unresponsive. Infants and children do not respond in the same manner as adults. For these young patients, how they respond to the environment and their parents is the best gauge of consciousness.

3. *Airway status.* This is a vitally important portion of the survey. If the patient is responsive determine if the patient can speak. If so, is the airway patent? Unresponsive patients will require that you open the airway. The procedures for this vary by the nature of the patient's condition. Opening the airway of a trauma patient will require you to use the jaw thrust method to prevent worsening any existing spinal injuries. For unresponsive medical patients, the head-tilt chin-lift may be used. The airway must then be inspected and cleared if necessary using suction and/or finger sweeps.

4. *Assess breathing.* Assessing breathing requires a careful examination of the patient. Responsive patients may still have extreme difficulty breathing. Look at the respiratory rate, depth, and the work required to breathe. For responsive patients, the ability to speak in full sentences is an important sign. In the unresponsive patient, look, listen, and feel for breathing. Ventilate if necessary. This includes ventilating patients who have some respiratory activity but are not breathing adequately. Inadequate breathing may be determined by very fast or very slow respiratory rates, increased effort of breathing, decreased or absent chest movement, and the lack of breath sounds or absence of breath sounds over one lung.

5. *Assess circulation.* This is done by assessing the patient's pulse and looking for major bleeding. For an responsive adult, assess the radial pulse. If the adult is unresponsive, the carotid pulse should be used. In children who are responsive, assess the brachial or radial pulse. In children who are unresponsive the curriculum recommends assessing the carotid or femoral pulse. In infants the brachial pulse is recommended regardless of the patient's level of consciousness. You will also assess the patient's skin color and temperature. Identifying major bleeding during the initial assessment is important since heavy bleeding can lead rapidly to death.

6. *Preliminary report to responding EMS units.* After completing the initial assessment you have an idea of your patient's complaints and their priority. Advising EMS units of this information while they are en route to the scene will allow them to prepare for the call and respond with the appropriate equipment. Advise the EMS units of the patient's age and gender, chief complaint, level of responsiveness, and the status of airway, breathing, and circulation. You may ask the incoming unit or units their estimated time of arrival (ETA).

The *First Responder physical exam* is the next step in your patient assessment. This is a special exam that has been developed to help First Responders locate and begin the initial management of the patient. The First Responder physical exam immediately follows the initial assessment. The actual scope of the examination would depend on the extent and severity of the patient's condition. The patient who has a simple cut finger would not require the entire examination. The patient who has fallen from a considerable height or is unresponsive and unable to provide a complaint would warrant full examination. You will also note a variation from trauma patients to medical patients. The medical patient will not require a detailed hands-on assessment of the entire body; rather, a majority of the information will come from the history taking. Therefore, when treating a patient with a medical complaint, the history may be performed before the physical examination.

The First Responder physical exam consists of examining the following body regions by inspecting (looking) and palpating (feeling):

1. Head

2. Neck

3. Chest

4. Abdomen

5. Pelvis

6. All four Extremities

You are inspecting and palpating for the following signs of injury:

- **D**eformities

- **O**pen injuries

- **T**enderness

- **S**welling

The mnemonic DOTS will help you to remember the signs to look for. You will notice that the areas of the body that you will examine are presented in a logical order. You should always assess in that same order. There will be times where there are obvious, grotesque injuries that could easily distract you from more serious problems. The assessment is basically in head-to-toe order. Following this order on every patient is one step in assuring that your assessment is accurate and thorough each time.

The *history* is a series of questions that is designed to develop pertinent medical information from the patient or the patient's family. SAMPLE is a mnemonic used to identify the parts of the history-taking process.

- *Signs and symptoms.* The chief complaint is usually the answer to the question "Why did you call EMS today?" This is usually the beginning of the history-taking process. Signs are conditions or changes to the patient that can be seen by the First

Responder. Examples of a sign are swelling around an injury or observing bleeding. Symptoms are feelings or conditions described by the patient. An example of a symptom is pain. Actual pain cannot be seen by the First Responder (although the patient's response to the pain may be obvious).

- *Allergies.* Determine if the patient has allergies to anything. This includes medication allergies as well as allergies to food and the environment.

- *Medications.* The medications that a patient takes or has taken in the past can tell you a lot about the person's medical conditions. Remember to ask about prescription and non-prescription medications that are taken currently or used in the recent past.

- *Pertinent past history.* This section of the history taking is very important. You are looking for past or current medical conditions that are pertinent to your care of the patient. You should determine if the patient is seeing a doctor for anything, if they have ever been hospitalized (this gives a clue to serious conditions or surgeries), along with asking about prior illnesses and injuries.

- *Last oral intake.* Ask the patient the last time that he or she has had anything to eat or drink. Determine the approximate time and the amount and type of food or drink.

- *Events leading up to the illness or injury.* It is important to know what led up to the patient's current condition. If you ask questions such as "What were you doing when this happened?" you will develop important information. Some trauma calls also involve medical conditions. This occurs when a patient loses consciousness and falls. You receive the call for a patient who fell. It is up to you to investigate the events leading up to the fall to find that your trauma patient has a medical problem, too.

The *ongoing assessment* is the final step in the patient assessment process. In some cases, such as when the additional EMS units arrive rapidly, you may not have time to get into the ongoing assessment. Care of the patient must be continued after the First Responder physical examination and history taking. This is the purpose of the ongoing assessment. This steps of this assessment include:

1. *Repeating the initial assessment.* The initial assessment is repeated at least every 5 minutes for an unstable patient and every

15 minutes for a stable patient. It is important to remember that patients may deteriorate during your care. You must reassess the mental status, airway, breathing, circulation and skin color, and temperature frequently. Be prepared to provide basic life support if necessary.

2. *Repeating the first responder physical examination* (if needed and if time permits).

3. *Monitoring interventions.* Any treatments or care that you have given the patient should be reassessed. Interventions are discussed later in this manual.

4. *Continuing to calm and reassure the patient.*

5. *Providing a "hand-off" report.* When the EMS personnel who are going to assume care of the patient arrive, you must brief them on the patient's condition. This is called a hand-off report. The report consists of:
   a. Age and gender
   b. Chief complaint
   c. Level of responsiveness
   d. Airway, breathing, and circulation status
   e. Physical findings
   f. Information obtained in the SAMPLE history
   g. Interventions provided and their effect on patient condition

The patient assessment process is an important one. Any care or interventions that you undertake with a patient depend on it.

REVIEW QUESTIONS

1. Which of the following is not a part of the scene size-up?
   A. Airway, breathing, and circulation
   B. Body substance isolation
   C. Mechanism of injury
   D. Determining how many patients are involved

2. Which of the following items would be addressed in the scene size-up?
   A. AVPU
   B. Opening the airway
   C. Brief radio report
   D. Calling for specialized units when required

3. Which of the following is not a mechanism of injury?
   A. A fall of 15 feet
   B. Chest trauma from a steering wheel
   C. Chest pain
   D. A broken arm from falling off a bicycle

4. The mechanism of injury may be determined from:
   A. the patient.
   B. observations of the scene.
   C. information from bystander witnesses.
   D. all of the above.

5. Nature of illness is the:
   A. reason that EMS was called for a medical patient.
   B. reason that EMS was called for a trauma patient.
   C. physical forces involved in the injury.
   D. same as the general impression.

6. Triage is a:
   A. system of sorting patients by treatment priority.
   B. step in the First Responder physical assessment.
   C. technique performed only by EMT-Paramedics.
   D. step in history taking.

7. It is important to determine the number of patients early because:
   A. it is important for statistical reasons.
   B. hospitals must be informed before the patient assessment.
   C. some of the patients may be children.
   D. once patient care has begun, you will be less likely to call for help.

8. The purpose of the initial assessment is to:
   A. call for additional resources.
   B. determine scene safety.
   C. identify and treat immediate threats to life.
   D. perform a head-to-toe examination.

9. The components of the general impression include:
   A. pulse, respirations, skin temperature, and color.
   B. the AVPU and SAMPLE history.
   C. the First Responder physical examination.
   D. assessment of the scene, chief complaint, and the age and gender of the patient.

10. The mnemonic used to remember the various levels of consciousness (unresponsiveness) is:
    A. AMPLE
    B. SAMPLE
    C. DOTS
    D. AVPU

11. In reference to assessing the level of consciousness of a young child, which statement is true?
    A. Children generally respond the same as adults.
    B. Attention should be paid to the child's interaction with parents and the environment.
    C. It is not possible to evaluate a young child's level of consciousness.
    D. None of the above.

12. During the airway assessment of a trauma patient with suspected spine injury the airway is opened using the:
    A. head-tilt chin lift.
    B. Sellick's maneuver.
    C. jaw thrust.
    D. none of the above

13. Which of the following is not part of the circulation check in the initial assessment?
    A. Looking for major bleeding
    B. Checking skin color and temperature
    C. Chief complaint
    D. Assessing the patient's pulse

14. The parts of the patient assessment, in order, are:
    A. size-up, initial assessment, history, ongoing assessment, First Responder physical exam.
    B. initial assessment, size-up, history, ongoing assessment, First Responder physical exam.
    C. size-up, initial assessment, First Responder physical exam, history, ongoing assessment.
    D. ongoing assessment, size-up, initial assessment, First Responder physical exam, history.

15. The DOTS mnemonic stands for:
    A. disability, open injuries, trauma, seizures.
    B. deformities, open injuries, tenderness, swelling.

C. dizziness, obstetrics, trauma, seizures.

D. deformities, open injuries, tenderness, seizures.

16. The First Responder physical assessment for an adult is generally performed in which order?

A. Head to toe

B. Toe to Head

C. Starting with obvious injuries first

D. Randomly to prevent anticipation by the patient

17. For medical patients, the SAMPLE history may be completed before the First Responder physical exam.

A. True

B. False

18. The SAMPLE mnemonic stands for:

A. seizures, altered mental status, medical emergencies, pain, last meal, and epilepsy.

B. signs, asthma, medications, pulse, last oral intake, events.

C. signs and symptoms, allergies, medications, past history, last oral intake, events.

D. none of the above.

19. Which of the following is not part of the hand-off report?

A. Age and gender of the patient

B. Blood pressure

C. Circulation status

D. Interventions provided

20. The difference between a sign and a symptom is that:

A. signs are found only in trauma patients.

B. symptoms are things that can be seen, signs are not.

C. signs are things that can be seen, symptoms are not.

D. there is no difference between the two terms.

21. When asking a patient about possible allergies you should ask about:

A. medication allergies only.

B. medication and food allergies only.

C. medication, food, and environmental allergies.

D. nothing; allergies are not a pertinent part of the history.

22. Which question best asks about the events leading up to a patient's illness or injury?
    A. What were you doing when this happened?
    B. Do you have any medical problems?
    C. Are you seeing a doctor for anything?
    D. Why did you call for EMS today?

23. Updating the incoming EMS units via radio will help them to prepare for patient care. This is usually done at the end of the:
    A. scene size-up.
    B. initial assessment.
    C. First Responder physical exam.
    D. ongoing assessment.

24. A patient with an isolated minor injury would not require the entire First Responder physical exam.
    A. True
    B. False

25. During the ongoing assessment patients must be reassessed at least every:
    A. 5 minutes for unstable patients, 15 minutes for stable patients.
    B. 15 minutes for unstable patients, 5 minutes for stable patients.
    C. 15 minutes for either stable or unstable.
    D. 10 minutes for unstable patients, 20 minutes for stable patients.

26. Which of the following steps is not part of the ongoing assessment?
    A. A check of interventions performed
    B. Retaking the entire history
    C. Reassessing mental status
    D. Reassessing pulse rate and quality

27. Inadequate breathing may be determined by all of the following except:
    A. effort or work of breathing.
    B. respiratory rate.
    C. looking, listening, and feeling.
    D. level of consciousness.

28. A patient has fallen from a ladder. He responds verbally but is confused. There are at least two trained First Responders at the scene. Of the following choices, which would be done first?
   A. Stabilize the spine.
   B. Check for deformities, open injuries, tenderness, and swelling.
   C. Assess the patient's breathing.
   D. Update incoming units with a radio report.

29. A patient who will respond when you speak but does not know where he is would be classified as _____ on the AVPU scale.
   A. alert
   B. verbal
   C. pain
   D. unresponsive

30. A complaint of dizziness would best be described as a:
   A. sign.
   B. symptom.
   C. disease.
   D. general impression.

ANSWERS WITH RATIONALE

1. A. Of the choices listed, body substance isolation, mechanism of injury determination, and determining the number of patients are all a part of the size-up. Airway, breathing, and circulation are part of the initial assessment, not the size-up.

2. D. Calling for specialized units is a part of the scene size-up. It is important to size up the scene thoroughly before beginning patient care. It has been shown that EMS personnel are less likely to call for the required help once they begin patient care.

3. C. Chest pain is a symptom and a nature of illness but is not a mechanism of injury. Mechanism of injury is used only in traumatic injury and should reflect a physical force. The other choices—a fall of 15 feet, chest trauma from the steering wheel, and the broken arm from falling off a bicycle—all involve trauma and physical forces.

4. D. The mechanism of injury may be determined from all of the choices listed. The patient, your observations of the scene,

and bystanders are all important sources of information. All three may not be available on every call, but each should be used when possible.

5. A. Nature of illness is a concept applied to medical patients. It is usually answered by determining why EMS was called. For example, if a patient requested EMS because of abdominal pain, the nature of illness would be "abdominal pain." This is similar to the chief complaint.

6. A. Triage is a system of sorting patients by treatment priority. Triage is used when there are more patients than the system can currently handle, usually at multiple-casualty incidents (MCIs). This allows the resources at hand to be used on those patients who can use it the most. This is discussed in greater detail in Chapter 14.

7. D. Proper care of a patient requires concentration and energy. Once you begin the patient care process it would be easy to lose track of other parts of the scene. This is why it is important to request any additional personnel or resources before beginning patient care. As stated earlier, providers are less likely to call for help once they begin patient care.

8. C. The initial assessment deals with immediate threats to life only. This includes airway, breathing and circulation. These problems must be identified *and* treated during the initial assessment. Scene safety and calling for resources should be completed before beginning the initial assessment. The head-to-toe examination is completed as part of the First Responder physical examination, which is performed after the initial assessment.

9. D. The general impression includes your assessment of the scene, the patient's chief complaint, and the age and gender of the patient. These items help you to form an impression of the scene. This impression will help you to determine further actions based on what you see and how serious you feel the patient's condition is.

10. D. The levels of consciousness that you will observe in the field are alert, verbal, pain, and unresponsive. These form the mnemonic AVPU. SAMPLE and AMPLE represent points in history taking. DOTS is used to remember what you will look for in the head-to-toe examination.

11. B. Children are not the same as adults. There are even differences between children of different ages. At a relatively young age, infants will recognize their parents. Failing to do this may indicate a decreased level of consciousness. The same goes for your

presence. Most infants and children would be upset and scared at the presence of a stranger, especially an EMS person with the need to examine the child with equipment that is sure to be perceived as scary. A lack of interest in the environment or failing to be apprehensive about you as a stranger could indicate a change in the level of consciousness. Of course, some children are not upset by strangers. Compare the everyday state of the child against their current state by asking the parents.

12. C. When a patient has a spine injury or the potential for a spine injury, the jaw thrust method is used to open the airway. Since the head is not tilted when performing the jaw thrust method, you will not worsen any existing spinal injuries.

13. C. The circulation step involves making sure that the patient has a pulse and determining whether blood is being sent to the body without problems. This would include looking for major bleeding and assessing the patient's pulse. Checking skin color and temperature is also important since reduced blood flow often causes cool, moist skin. The chief complaint is obtained upon your arrival at the scene and during the general impression.

14. C. The parts of the patient assessment, in order, are: scene size-up, initial assessment, First Responder physical exam, history, and ongoing assessment. This question also brings up a test-taking point. Some may argue that the history may be taken before completing the First Responder physical exam when dealing with medical patients. Although this is true, it does not change the fact that there are only four choices and you must choose the *best* answer of what is given. What should help you choose C as the correct answer is that none of the other answers are close to correct. Both A and B list the ongoing assessment before the First Responder physical exam, which is clearly wrong. Choice D lists the ongoing assessment first. Since the ongoing assessment is the last step, your knowledge of the patient assessment steps, with some careful reading will help you choose the correct answer.

15. B. DOTS stands for deformities, open injuries, tenderness, and swelling. This question requires careful reading, since some of the incorrect answers are very close.

16. A. When assessing an adult the physical exam is generally performed in a head-to-toe order. It is important to perform the assessment in a logical order each time so that injuries and conditions are not missed. Avoid focusing on obvious or grotesque injuries. These could cause you to ignore more important but hidden life-threatening problems.

17. A. Patients who have suffered traumatic injuries require a physical exam geared toward the trauma they have experienced. When examining a medical patient, a majority of your information will be obtained from your SAMPLE history. There will be less to look for in a hands-on exam of a medical patient. Therefore, it is acceptable and often advisable to perform the history before the physical exam for medical patients.

18. C. SAMPLE stands for signs and symptoms, allergies, medications, past history, last oral intake, and events. This mnemonic will help you to remember the components of the patient history.

19. B. The age and gender of the patient, circulation status, and interventions provided are all part of the hand-off report. Blood pressure taking is not included in the 1995 National Standard First Responder Curriculum and is therefore incorrect. This is another reminder about the influence of the curriculum on the National Registry First Responder Examination.

20. C. Signs are things that can be seen, symptoms are not. An example of a sign is a discoloration of the skin over a possible broken bone. A symptom is related by the patient. An example of a symptom is chest pain.

21. C. When asking about allergies, you should ask about medication, environmental, and food allergies. All three may affect the patient's condition.

22. A. Determining the events that lead up to the patient's condition is very important. The question "What were you doing when this happened?" is the best choice to determine the events. If you are treating a patient with injuries from a fall it is important to know whether the patient tripped and fell or passed out and fell to the ground. For chest pain patients it is important to know what the patient was doing when the pain came on. It is important to distinguish whether the patient was resting or exerting himself and advise the EMS unit personnel who will continue care for the patient.

23. B. The radio report to update responding EMS units is made after the initial assessment. It is at this point that you will have important information about the scene and the patient's airway, breathing, and circulation status to relay to incoming EMS units.

24. A. Patients with minor injuries that do not affect the entire body do not require the entire physical examination. A person who had cut his finger and has minor bleeding would not require a head-

to-toe exam. Many patients will require a full exam. If a person falls several feet from a ladder, he or she would receive the entire examination even if the person claimed minor injury since the mechanism of injury is such that other injuries could be possible.

25. A. During the ongoing examination unstable patients are reassessed at least every 5 minutes, while stable patients must be reassessed at least every 15 minutes.

26. B. During the ongoing assessment it is not necessary to retake the entire history from the patient. You will, however, repeat the initial assessment, determine the level of consciousness, and check any treatments or interventions that you have provided.

27. D. The effort or work of breathing, respiratory rate, and looking, listening, and feeling are all directly involved in determining whether the patient is breathing adequately. While a patient who is not breathing adequately may have an altered level of consciousness, it is not directly involved in breathing determination.

28. A. Spinal precautions must be considered and applied early in the call. You would have examined the mechanism of injury (fall from a ladder) during the size-up and determined that stabilization of the spine is necessary. In the case presented the patient is conscious and there is sufficient help present to stabilize the spine immediately. With the patient who is conscious, he may try to look around or otherwise move his head. And remember, if the patient requires airway care or ventilation, you or another First Responder would be required to maintain stabilization while caring for the airway.

29. B. The patient presented in this question responds to verbal stimulus. He is not alert because he does not know where he is. Since he does respond verbally, his level of responsiveness is above the P (pain) level.

30. B. Dizziness is a symptom. The sensation itself cannot be palpated or seen. Nausea is another example of a symptom. Nausea cannot be seen. Vomiting is a sign; it can be seen. A sign, such as a bruise, can be seen. A deformity to a bone can be seen and palpated. The basic difference between a sign and a symptom is that a symptom is something that is experienced by the patient. The patient will describe the symptom to you. A sign is something that can be observed by the First Responder.

LESSON

4-1 Circulation

D O T
OBJECTIVES

Cognitive Objectives

At the completion of this lesson, the First Responder student will be able to:

4-1.1 List the reasons for the heart to stop beating.

4-1.2 Define the components of cardiopulmonary resuscitation.

4-1.3 Describe each link in the chain of survival and how it relates to the EMS system.

4-1.4 List the steps of one-rescuer adult CPR.

4-1.5 Describe the technique of external chest compressions on an adult patient.

4-1.6 Describe the technique of external chest compressions on an infant.

4-1.7 Describe the technique of external chest compressions on a child.

4-1.8 Explain when the First Responder is able to stop CPR.

4-1.9 List the steps of two-rescuer adult CPR.

4-1.10 List the steps of infant CPR.

4-1.11 List the steps of child CPR.

Affective Objectives

At the completion of this lesson, the First Responder student will be able to:

4-1.12 Respond to the feelings that the family of a patient may be having during a cardiac event.

4-1.13 Demonstrate a caring attitude towards patients with cardiac events who request emergency medical services.

4-1.14 Place the interests of the patient with a cardiac event as the foremost consideration when making any and all patient care decisions.

4-1.15 Communicate with empathy with family members and friends of the patient with a cardiac event.

Psychomotor Objectives

At the completion of this lesson, the First Responder student will be able to:

4-1.16 Demonstrate the proper technique of chest compressions on an adult.

4-1.17 Demonstrate the proper technique of chest compressions on a child.

4-1.18 Demonstrate the proper technique of chest compressions on an infant.

4-1.19 Demonstrate the steps of adult one-rescuer CPR.

4-1.20 Demonstrate the steps of adult two-rescuer CPR.

4-1.21 Demonstrate child CPR.

4-1.22 Demonstrate infant CPR.

QUICK REVIEW The circulatory system is responsible for delivering oxygen and nutrients to the tissues as well as removing waste products. The heart is a four-chambered muscular organ that is responsible for the circulation of blood. Each time the heart contracts, a quantity of blood is forced into the bloodstream, causing the pulse to be felt. When the heart for any reason stops beating, a pulse will no longer be felt. This may happen for many reasons. These reasons include:

- Heart disease and sudden death

- Respiratory problems, especially in infants and children

- Stroke, diabetes, allergic reactions, and other medical conditions

- Drowning, poisoning, electrical shock, and similar incidents

- Trauma and severe bleeding

When the heart stops, the First Responder must take immediate action and initiate CPR. CPR may be performed on any of the conditions listed above. Although there may be modifications to the way some of the procedures are performed, any patient in cardiac arrest may receive CPR. The alternative is death.

Cardiopulmonary resuscitation (CPR) is a procedure that combines artificial respiration and external chest compressions. CPR oxygenates and circulates blood since the heart has stopped. The external chest compressions of CPR change the pressure within the chest cavity and cause blood to flow from the heart. This is not nearly as effective as the heart's own activity and will sustain life only for a short period of time. CPR is necessary, but it is only one link of a chain of survival required to save the patient.

The chain of survival consists of four "links." Each link is required to give a patient the maximum chance of survival. The links are:

- *Early access*. The EMS system must be alerted so that the remaining steps fall into place. Each of the links in the chain of survival relies on the others. If one link is weak or fails, the patient's chances of survival are greatly reduced. In keeping with this early access link, rapid recognition of a cardiac emergency and phoning immediately for help is essential.

- *Early CPR*. Early CPR is required to circulate the oxygenated blood to keep tissues alive so that the patient will be responsive to the next link in the chain. CPR may be performed by bystanders and family members as well as First Responders.

- *Early defibrillation*. The earlier that defibrillation can be performed, the better. Defibrillation is taught to EMT-Bs and some First Responders. This has been identified as one of the single most important factors in patient survival.

- *Early advanced care*. The patient requires access to advanced life support from EMT-Intermediates, Paramedics, and hospital personnel.

Cardiopulmonary Resuscitation

CPR consists of chest compressions and rescue breathing. The chest compressions are performed over the lower half of the sternum. The depth of compression varies by the age of the patient.

- Infant (birth to 1 year): 1/2 to 1 inch

- Child (1 to 8 years): 1 to 1 1/2 inches

- Adult (over 8 years): 1 1/2 to 2 inches

One-rescuer adult CPR

1. Establish unresponsiveness.

2. Activate the EMS system.

3. Open the airway using the head-tilt chin-lift or jaw thrust for trauma patients.

4. Check for breathing. If absent,

5. Give two slow breaths (1 1/2 to 2 seconds each), allowing for exhalation between breaths.

6. Check carotid pulse.

7. If no pulse, provide compressions at ratio of 15 compressions to 2 ventilations at the rate of 80 to 100 per minute followed by two slow breaths.

8. Check pulse after four cycles of 15:2.

9. If required, begin again with chest compressions.

Two-rescuer adult CPR

1. Establish unresponsiveness.

2. Activate the EMS system.

   Rescuer 1

3. Open the airway using the head-tilt chin-lift or jaw thrust for trauma patients.

4. Give two slow breaths (1 1/2 to 2 seconds each), allowing for exhalation between breaths.

5. Check carotid pulse.

6. If no pulse, begin compressions. Rescuer 2 would perform five chest compressions at the rate of 80 to 100 per minute, then rescuer 1 would perform one slow breath.

7. After 1 minute of CPR, check the carotid pulse.

8. If required, continue CPR at the 5:1 ratio.

Infant CPR

1. Establish unresponsiveness. If a second rescuer is present, activate the EMS system.

2. Open the airway using the head-tilt chin-lift or jaw thrust for trauma.

3. Check for breathing (look, listen, feel).

4. If breathing is absent, give two slow breaths 1 to 1 1/2 seconds per breath. Watch for chest rise with each breath and allow for exhalation.

5. Check the brachial pulse.

6. If the pulse is absent, perform five compressions and one slow ventilation. The compressions are at a rate of at least 100 per minute. Repeat this cycle.

7. After about 1 minute of CPR, check the brachial pulse. If you are alone, stop and activate the EMS system, then continue CPR if necessary

Child CPR

1. Establish unresponsiveness. If a second rescuer is present, activate the EMS system.

2. Open the airway using the head-tilt chin-lift or jaw thrust for trauma.

3. Check for breathing (look, listen, feel).

4. If breathing is absent, give two slow breaths 1 to 1 1/2 seconds per breath. Watch for chest rise with each breath and allow for exhalation.

5. Check the carotid pulse.

6. If the pulse is absent, perform five compressions and one slow ventilation. The compressions are at a rate of 100 per minute. Repeat this cycle.

7. After about 1 minute of CPR, check the brachial pulse. If you are alone, stop and activate the EMS system, then continue CPR if necessary.

In all of the patients listed above, if a pulse returns but breathing is still absent, discontinue compressions but continue rescue breathing. These slow breaths are given once every 3 seconds for infants and children (20/minute) and every 5 seconds (12/minute) for adults. Monitor the pulse so that compressions may be restarted if necessary. CPR must be continued until one of several things happens:

- You turn the patient over to another qualified person (another First Responder, EMT-B, or hospital personnel).

- The patient regains a pulse (rescue breathing may still be needed).

- A physician pronounces the patient dead.

- You are physically exhausted and cannot continue.

REVIEW QUESTIONS

1. The circulatory system is responsible for:
   A. delivering oxygen to the tissues.
   B. removing waste products from the tissues.
   C. delivering nutrients to the tissues.
   D. all of the above.

2. Which of the following is not part of the chain of survival?
   A. Early access
   B. Early prudent heart living
   C. Early CPR
   D. Early advanced care

3. Which of the following may cause the heart to stop beating?
   A. Heart attack
   B. Stroke
   C. Allergic reaction
   D. All of the above

4. Which of the following statements about CPR is false?
   A. CPR must be started as early as possible.
   B. CPR will sustain life indefinitely.

C. CPR increases the amount of time that defibrillation will be effective.

D. CPR is a combination of ventilations and chest compressions.

5. After performing the initial look, listen, and feel for breathing, you find that your patient does not have any respirations. Your next step is to:

A. check the pulse.

B. administer two quick breaths.

C. administer two slow breaths.

D. begin chest compressions.

6. Which of the following statements about cardiopulmonary resuscitation is false?

A. CPR combines artificial ventilation and chest compressions.

B. CPR alone has a better chance of saving a patient than do CPR and early defibrillation.

C. CPR may be performed on patients of any age.

D. CPR may be performed on a pulseless patient with chest injuries.

7. Patients who are in cardiac arrest and require CPR must be placed

A. in the recovery position.

B. supine on a soft surface to prevent injury.

C. supine on a firm surface.

D. prone on a firm surface.

8. The proper location to perform a pulse check on an unresponsive adult is the:

A. brachial.

B. femoral.

C. carotid.

D. posterior tibial.

9. When performing rescue breathing on an adult patient, each breath should be given over _____ seconds.

A. 1/2 to 3/4

B. 1 to 2

C. 1 1/2 to 2

D. 2 to 4

10. Which of the following choices lists the steps of CPR in the most proper sequence?
    A. Activate the EMS system, check carotid pulse, provide ventilations, provide compressions.
    B. Establish unresponsiveness, activate the EMS system, open the airway, check for breathing.
    C. Provide two slow ventilations, check for breathing, provide compressions.
    D. Establish unresponsiveness, activate the EMS system, check carotid pulse, check breathing.

11. After CPR has begun, pulses should be checked:
    A. every 5 minutes.
    B. after each 15:2 cycle.
    C. every minute.
    D. after about 1 minute and then every few minutes thereafter.

12. The most common cause of cardiac arrest in infants and young children is:
    A. respiratory problems.
    B. heart attack.
    C. electrocution.
    D. none of the above.

13. What is the correct compression depth for infant CPR?
    A. 1/2 to 1 inch
    B. 1 to 1 1/2 inch
    C. 1 1/2 to 2 inches
    D. None of the above

14. What is the correct compression depth for CPR on a child?
    A. 1/2 to 3/4 inch
    B. 1 to 1 1/2 inches
    C. 1 1/2 to 2 inches
    D. None of the above

15. What is the correct compression depth for CPR on an adult?
    A. 1/2 to 1 inch
    B. 1 to 1 1/2 inches
    C. 1 1/2 to 2 inches
    D. 2 to 4 inches

16. The ratio of compressions to ventilations for infant and child CPR is:
    A. 15 compressions to 1 ventilation.
    B. 15 compressions to 2 ventilations.
    C. 5 compressions to 1 ventilation.
    D. 5 compressions to 2 ventilations.

17. The ratio of compressions to ventilations for adult one-rescuer CPR is:
    A. 15 compressions to 1 ventilation.
    B. 15 compressions to 2 ventilations.
    C. 5 compressions to 1 ventilation.
    D. 5 compressions to 2 ventilations.

18. If you are alone and caring for an infant in respiratory arrest, you should:
    A. activate the EMS system immediately.
    B. perform rescue breathing for 1 minute and then activate the EMS system.
    C. perform rescue breathing until breathing resumes, then contact EMS.
    D. perform rescue breathing for 3 to 5 minutes, then contact EMS.

19. After performing CPR for 1 minute, your adult patient regains a pulse but has no respirations. You should:
    A. continue administering rescue breathing at the rate of 12 per minute.
    B. continue administering rescue breathing at the rate of 20 per minute.
    C. continue chest compressions and ventilations.
    D. place the patient in the recovery position.

20. The First Responder may discontinue CPR in all of the following situations except when the:
    A. First Responder is physically exhausted and unable to continue.
    B. patient regains a pulse.
    C. patient is turned over to another qualified person.
    D. family feels that CPR would only prolong suffering.

1. D. All of the answers are correct. The circulatory system delivers oxygen, removes waste products, and delivers nutrients. These items are transported by the blood to and from all parts of the body.

2. B. Prudent heart living (maintaining a heart-healthy lifestyle) is not a part of the chain of survival. The chain of survival refers to actions or parts of the system that are activated in the event of an actual cardiac emergency.

3. D. All of the answers listed could cause the heart to stop beating. Heart attacks damage heart muscle, a severe stroke can also cause the heart to stop beating. Allergic reactions may be severe and cause airway problems and shock which lead to cardiac arrest.

4. B. CPR must be started as early as possible, increases the amount of time that a shock will be effective in restoring a heart rhythm, and is a combination of ventilations and compressions. CPR will not sustain life indefinitely. CPR is only a small percentage as effective as the heart's own beating.

5. C. Once you find that the patient isn't breathing you will breath for him or her by giving two slow breaths. This will be followed by a pulse check. You would not begin chest compressions until you determine they are needed by checking the pulse.

6. B. As noted in an earlier question, CPR will not sustain life indefinitely. It is best when used as a short-term measure to make defibrillation more likely to work. This makes choice B false. CPR with early defibrillation is an ideal combination.

7. C. A patient who requires CPR must be placed supine (on the back) and on a firm surface. It would not be possible to do compressions on a patient in the recovery position or prone. Compressions would be ineffective if performed on a soft surface such as a bed.

8. C. The carotid pulse would be used when checking an unresponsive adult patient.

9. C. When performing rescue breathing or ventilating during CPR, ventilations are given to an adult patient slowly, over 1 1/2 to 2 seconds each. This should allow for air to exit the patient before giving the next breath.

10. B. Choice B provides the proper sequence among the choices listed. Questions such as this require careful reading. You will

note that some choices are similar and could easily be chosen without careful consideration.

11. D. Once CPR has begun, pulses should be checked after the first minute and every few minutes thereafter. One minute is four cycles of 15:2.

12. A. Young children do not suffer heart attacks as adults do. Although these patients may be electrocuted, respiratory problems are by far the most common cause of cardiac arrest in children. This highlights the importance of airway care for infants and children!

13. A. The chest of the infant receiving CPR is compressed 1/2 to 1 inch.

14. B. The correct compression depth for child CPR is 1 to 1 1/2 inches.

15. C. The correct compression depth for adult CPR is 1 1/2 to 2 inches. You will note that the compression depths from infant to adult are sequential: 1/2 to 1 for infants, 1 to 1 1/2 for children, and 1 1/2 to 2 for adults.

16. C. CPR for infants and children differs from that for adults in many ways. One of these ways is that the compression-to-ventilation ratio for both one- and two-rescuer infant and child CPR is 5:1.

17. B. The compression-to-ventilation ratio for adult one-rescuer CPR is 15 compressions to 2 ventilations.

18. B. If you are alone and performing CPR or rescue breathing on an infant, you would perform CPR or rescue breathing for 1 minute and then activate the EMS system. Remember that the main cause of cardiac arrest in infants and children are respiratory problems. This is why 1 minute of care might make a difference by opening the airway and providing ventilations and/or CPR.

19. A. There will be occasions when the pulse will return but respirations do not (or respirations are very shallow and not enough to support life). In this case you must continue rescue breathing until adequate respirations return or another qualified person takes over care of the patient.

20. D. Choices A to C are correct. Each indicates a situation where a First Responder could discontinue CPR. Without a do not resuscitate (DNR) order, the family could not request that care be withheld or discontinued.

5-1 Medical Emergencies

DOT OBJECTIVES

Cognitive Objectives

At the completion of this lesson, the First Responder student will be able to:

5-1.1 Identify the patient with a general medical complaint.

5-1.2 Explain the steps in providing emergency medical care to a patient with a general medical complaint.

5-1.3 Identify the patient who presents with a specific medical complaint of altered medical status.

5-1.4 Explain the steps in providing emergency medical care to a patient with an altered mental status.

5-1.5 Identify the patient who presents with a specific medical complaint of seizures.

5-1.6 Explain the steps in providing emergency medical care to a patient with seizures.

5-1.7 Identify the patient who presents with a specific medical complaint of exposure to cold.

5-1.8 Explain the steps in providing emergency medical care to a patient with an exposure to cold.

5-1.9 Identify the patient who presents with a specific medical complaint of exposure to heat.

5-1.10 Explain the steps in providing emergency medical care to a patient with an exposure to heat.

5-1.11 Identify the patient who presents with a specific medical complaint of behavioral change.

5-1.12 Explain the steps in providing emergency medical care to a patient with a behavioral change.

5-1.13 Identify the patient who presents with a specific complaint of a psychological crisis.

5-1.14 Explain the steps in providing emergency medical care to a patient with psychological crisis.

Affective Objectives

At the completion of this lesson, the First Responder student will be able to:

5-1.15 Attend to the feelings of the patient and/or family when dealing with the patient with a general medical complaint.

5-1.16 Attend to the feelings of the patient and/or family when dealing with the patient with a specific medical complaint.

5-1.17 Explain the rationale for modifying your behavior toward the patient with a behavioral emergency.

5-1.18 Demonstrate a caring attitude towards patients with a general medical complaint who request emergency medical services.

5-1.19 Place the interests of the patient with a general medical complaint as the foremost consideration when making any and all patient care decisions.

5-1.20 Communicate with empathy to patient with a general medical complaint, as well as with family members and friends of the patient.

5-1.21 Demonstrate a caring attitude towards patients with a specific medical complaint who request emergency medical services.

5-1.22 Place the interests of the patient with a specific medical complaint as the foremost consideration when making any and all a patient care decisions.

5-1.23 Communicate with empathy to patients with a specific medical complaint, as well as with family members and friends of the patient.

5-1.24 Demonstrate a caring attitude towards patients with a behavioral problem who request emergency medical services.

5-1.25 Place the interests of the patient with a behavioral problem as the foremost consideration when making any and all patient care decisions.

5-1.26 Communicate with empathy to patients with a behavioral problem, as well as with family members and friends of the patient.

Psychomotor Objectives

At the completion of this lesson, the First Responder student will be able to:

5-1.27 Demonstrate the steps in providing emergency medical care to a patient with a general medical complaint.

5-1.28 Demonstrate the steps in providing emergency medical care to a patient with an altered mental status.

5-1.29 Demonstrate the steps in providing emergency medical care to a patient with seizures.

5-1.30 Demonstrate the steps in providing emergency medical care to a patient with an exposure to cold.

5-1.31 Demonstrate the steps in providing emergency medical care to a patient with an exposure to heat.

5-1.32 Demonstrate the steps in providing emergency medical care to a patient with a behavioral change.

5-1.33 Demonstrate the steps in providing emergency medical care to a patient with a psychological crisis.

QUICK REVIEW The patient with a general medical complaint, such as dizziness, nausea, headache, and shortness of breath, is very common in most EMS systems. The First Responder must provide assessment and treatment of patients with general medical complaints by providing the following: a scene size-up prior to initiating emergency medical care, an initial assessment, a physical exam as required by the patient's complaint, and an ongoing assessment as needed while waiting for other EMS resources to arrive on the scene. Specific medical complaints discussed in this chapter include: altered medical status, seizures, exposure to cold or heat, and behavioral problems. Additional (optional) information on medical complaints is covered in the final chapter.

Some patients present with an altered mental status that is defined as a sudden or gradual decrease in the patient's level of responsiveness and understanding ranging from disorientation to unresponsiveness. There are many reasons for an altered level of consciousness, some of which are: fever, infections, poisoning (drugs/alcohol/toxic substances), low blood sugar, head injury, decreased levels of oxygen to the brain (hypoxia), and psychiatric conditions.

Your focus as a First Responder should be to support the patient using lifesaving measures and maintaining scene safety. It is not imperative that the First Responder determine the cause of the altered mental status. In some instances this may be difficult even for the physician in the emergency department to determine without sophisticated tests.

The steps in providing emergency medical care to the patient with an altered mental status include a complete:

1. Scene size-up

2. Initial assessment

3. Physical exam as required by the patient's condition or complaint

4. Ongoing assessment

5. Attempt to comfort, calm, and reassure the patient while awaiting additional EMS resources

The period of altered mental status may be brief or prolonged. It is important for the First Responder to remember that the patient with an altered mental status may not be able to protect his or her airway from foreign materials. Evaluate the need for airway adjuncts such as an OPA or NPA and bag-valve-mask or pocket mask ventilation assistance or supplemental oxygen. The unresponsive nontraumatic patient should be placed in the recovery position. Do not give anything by mouth or place anything in the patient's mouth, other than an OPA, and have the suction unit nearby.

Some patients present with the specific medical complaint of seizures, which are sudden attacks usually related to nervous system function. There are many types of seizures, which are caused by such reasons as chronic medical conditions such as epilepsy, fever, infections, poisoning from drugs, alcohol or other toxins, low blood sugar, head injury, decreased levels of oxygen (hypoxia), brain tumors, complications of pregnancy, and other unknown causes.

It is the First Responder's responsibility to support the seizure patient, providing lifesaving care and emotional support. It is not the First Responder's responsibility to determine the cause of the seizure. Some seizures produce violent muscle contractions and convulsions. They usually last less for than 5 minutes, but they may be prolonged. The patients are usually unresponsive and may vomit during the convulsion. After the seizure the patients are very tired and want to sleep. Seizures rarely are life threatening but should be considered a serious emergency.

The steps in providing emergency medical care for a patient with seizures include:

1. Providing a complete scene size-up, initial assessment on all patients, physical exam as required by the patient's condition or complaint, and ongoing assessment.

2. Assure that the airway is patent and place the patient in the recovery position if there is not a possibility of a spine injury. Never restrain the patient or place anything in a patient's mouth. Have the suction unit available at the patient's side, and if the patient is bluish or cyanotic, assure an open airway and assist ventilations with supplemental oxygen.

3. Comfort, calm, and reassure the patient while awaiting additional EMS resources. Protect the patient from the environment and protect their modesty by asking bystanders to leave the area.

4. Be sure to report your assessment findings to the arriving EMS unit. If you observe and can describe the seizure duration and actions of the patient to arriving EMS units, you may be the only witness to the seizure and your description could be helpful in determining the cause of the seizure.

Remember the relationship of seizure management to airway management, in that seizure patients will have significant oral secretions. It will be essential that these patients be placed in the recovery position once the convulsion has ended. Patients who are actively seizing, bluish (cyanotic), and breathing inadequately should be ventilated with supplemental oxygen as soon as possible.

Some patients present with the specific medical complaint of an exposure to cold. Effects from cold exposure can have a generalized or local effect on the body. Factors that can contribute to generalized cold emergencies include:

- A cold environment (especially windy or wet)
- Very young or very old patients
- Patients with preexisting medical conditions that involve poor circulation
- Patients with alcohol or drugs

Generalized cold exposure is also called *hypothermia*. Patients with hypothermia will have the following signs and symptoms:

- Obvious exposure to a cold environment
- Subtle exposure combined with an underlying illness, overdose or poisoning, or a decreased ambient temperature, as in the home of an elderly person who is on a fixed income
- Cool/cold temperature as measured by the first responder by placing the back of the hand directly on the patient's abdomen
- Shivering
- Decreased mental status or motor function, which correlates with the degree of hypothermia (patients may have one or more of the following: poor coordination, memory disturbances and confusion, reduced touch sensation or loss of touch sensation, mood changes, patients becoming less communicative, dizziness, and speech difficulty)
- Stiff or rigid posture
- Muscular rigidity
- Poor judgment where a patient may actually remove clothing
- Complaints of joint or muscle stiffness

The steps in providing emergency medical care for a patient with hypothermia include:

1. Provide a complete scene size-up, initial assessment on all patients, physical exam as required by the patient's condition or complaint, and ongoing assessment.

2. Assess pulses for 30 to 45 seconds before starting CPR. Quickly remove the patient from the cold environment and protect him or her from further heat loss. If the patient has on wet clothing, remove the clothing and cover the patient with a blanket (top and bottom).

3. Be sure to handle the patient extremely gently, as rough handling can cause the patient to go into cardiac arrest from ventricular fibrillation. Do not allow the patient to walk or exert himself or herself. The patient should not receive anything by mouth, especially stimulants such as coffee, tea, or cigarettes, which can worsen the patient's condition. Do not massage the extremities.

4. Comfort, calm, and reassure the patient while awaiting for additional EMS resources. Protect the patient from the environment by covering with a blanket to keep him or her warm.

A patient may present with a local cold emergency such as freezing or near-freezing of a body part. This usually occurs in fingers, toes, the face, ears, and nose. The signs and symptoms of local cold injuries with clear demarcation depend on the stage of the injury (e.g., early or late). An *early* or *superficial cold injury* presents with:

- Blanching of the skin; palpation of the skin does not allow the color to return.

- There is loss of feeling and sensation in the injured area.

- The skin remains cold, yet soft.

- If rewarmed, the patient will have a tingling sensation.

    A *later* or *deep cold injury* presents with:

- Skin is white and waxy.

- Palpation yields a firm to frozen feeling.

- Swelling may be present.

- Blisters may be present.

- If thawed or partially thawed, the skin may appear flushed with areas of purple and blanching or may be mottled and cyanotic.

The steps in providing emergency medical care for a patient with a local cold injury include:

1. Provide a complete scene size-up, initial assessment on all patients, physical exam as required by the patient's condition or complaint, and ongoing assessment.

2. Remove the patient quickly from the cold environment and protect him or her from further heat loss. Protect the cold-injured extremity from further injury. If the patient has on wet clothing, remove the clothing and cover the patient with a blanket (top and bottom).

3. If the patient has an early or superficial injury, stabilize the extremity manually, cover it, and do not rub, massage, or reexpose to the cold.

4. If the patient has a late or deep cold injury, remove any jewelry and cover the area with dry clothing or dressings. *Do not* break blisters, rub or massage the area, apply heat, rewarm, or allow the patient to walk on the affected extremity.

5. Comfort, calm and reassure the patient while awaiting for additional EMS resources. Protect the patient from the environment by covering with a blanket to keep him or her warm.

Some patients present with the specific medical complaint of exposure to heat. Predisposing factors that can contribute to generalized heat emergencies include:

- A high ambient temperature, which reduces the body's ability to lose heat by radiation

- A high relative humidity, which reduces the body's ability to lose heat through evaporation

- Exercise and activity, which can cause the body to lose more than 1 liter of sweat per hour

- Patients who are very young or very old

- Preexisting illness and/or conditions

- Drugs and/or medications

Signs and symptoms of heat emergencies include the following:

- Muscular cramps

- Weakness or exhaustion

- Dizziness or faintness

- Rapid heart rate

- Mental status altered to unresponsive

The steps in providing emergency medical care for a patient with a heat exposure emergency include:

1. Provide a complete scene size-up, initial assessment on all patients, physical exam as required by the patient's condition or complaint, and ongoing assessment.

2. Remove the patient quickly from the hot environment and place him or her in a cool environment such as an air-conditioned room or ambulance. You can try to cool the patient by fanning, but this may be ineffective in high-humidity situations.

3. Comfort, calm, and reassure the patient while awaiting for additional EMS resources. Place the patient in the recovery position.

Some patients present with the specific medical complaint of a behavioral emergency. Behavior is the manner in which a person acts or performs, including any or all of a person's activities, including physical and mental activity. A behavioral emergency is a situation where the patient exhibits abnormal behavior that is unacceptable or intolerable to the patient, family, or community. This behavior can be due to extremes of emotion leading to violence or other inappropriate behavior, or can be due to a psychological or physical condition such as lack of oxygen (hypoxia) or low blood sugar (hypoglycemia).

Many general factors may alter a patient's behavior. Common causes for behavior alteration include:

- Situational stresses

- Illness or injury

- Low blood sugar

- Lack of oxygen

- Inadequate blood flow to the brain

- Head trauma

- Excessive cold

- Excessive heat

- Mind altering substances such as alcohol and drugs

- Psychiatric problems

- Psychological crises such as panic; agitation; bizarre thinking and behavior; danger to self or self-destructive behavior, such as suicide; and danger to others, such as threatening behavior or violence

When assessing a behavior emergency patient, keep in mind the following principles:

- Identify yourself and let the person know you are there to help.

- Inform the person of what you are doing.

- Ask questions in a calm, reassuring voice.

- Without being judgmental, allow the patient to describe what happened.

- Show that you are listening by rephrasing or repeating part of what is said.

- Acknowledge the patient's feelings.

- Assess the patient's mental status in terms of their appearance, activity, speech, and orientation for time, person, and place.

- Assess the potential for violence by taking into consideration your complete scene size-up; history of known aggression or combativeness from information provided by the family and/or bystanders; the patient's posture, which may threaten either the patient or others (i.e., clenched fists or lethal objects in hands); vocal activity such as yelling or verbally threatening harm to self or others; physical activity such as moving toward the caregiver; carrying heavy or threatening objects; tense muscles; or quick irregular movements.

The steps in providing emergency medical care for a patient with a behavioral emergency include:

1. Provide a complete scene size-up, initial assessment on all patients, physical exam as required by the patient's condition or complaint, and ongoing assessment.

2. Comfort, calm, and reassure the patient while awaiting additional EMS resources. Calm the patient and do not leave the person alone.

3. Consider the need for law enforcement, as some patients may be dangerous.

4. Turn medications or drugs found over to transporting EMS resources if the patient appears to have overdosed.

The First Responder should be aware of various methods available to calm a behavioral emergency patient:

- Acknowledge that the person seems upset and restate that you are there to help.

- Inform the person of what you are doing.

- Ask questions in a calm, reassuring voice.

- Maintain a comfortable distance, not invading the patient's personal space.

- Encourage the patient to state what is troubling him or her.

- Do not make any quick moves.

- Respond honestly to the patient's questions.

- Do not threaten, challenge, or argue with disturbed patients.

- Tell the truth; do not lie to the patient.

- Do not "play along" with visual or auditory disturbances of the patient.

- Involve trusted family members or friends.

- Be prepared to stay at the scene for a long time. Always remain with the patient.

- Avoid unnecessary physical contact. Call additional help if needed.

- Use good eye contact but do not stare at the patient.

In some situations it may be necessary to protect both the First Responder and the patient by actually restraining the patient. Restraint should be avoided unless the patient is a danger to his or her self or others. When using restraints, have the police present, and if possible, get approval from medical control. If restraints must be used, they should be humane and you should work in conjunction with the EMS providers.

Avoid using unreasonable force to restrain a patient. Reasonable force depends on what force is necessary to keep a patient from injuring himself or herself, or others. The reasonableness is determined by looking at all circumstances involved, such as: patient's size and strength, type of abnormal behavior, gender of the patient, mental state of the patient, and method of restraint to be used. Be aware that after a period of combativeness and aggression some apparently calm patients may cause unexpected and sudden injury to self and others. Avoid acts or physical force that may cause injury to a patient.

EMS personnel may use reasonable force to defend against attack by emotionally disturbed patients. Whenever possible, seek medical control involvement as well as police assistance, especially if during scene size-up the patient appears or acts aggressive or combative. First Responders should also be prepared to protect himself or herself against false accusations from a behavioral emergency patient. This is best done by documentation of abnormal behavior exhibited by the patient as objectively as possible. Have witnesses in attendance especially during transport. An emotionally disturbed patient may accuse First Responders of sexual misconduct. Make sure to have an EMS provider of the same gender and third-party witnesses.

Be knowledgeable of the medical/legal considerations of dealing with behavioral emergencies in your state and region. An emotionally disturbed patient who consents to care helps to decrease potential legal problems. If the patient resists treatment, consider the following:

- Emotionally disturbed patients will often resist treatment.

- Emotionally disturbed patients may threaten First Responders and others. You should have a high tolerance for verbal abuse, but you are never expected to take physical abuse from patients.

- To provide care against patient's will, you must have a reasonable belief that the patient would harm himself or herself, or others.

- If a threat to self or others, the patient may be transported without consent after you consult with medical control.

- Usually, law enforcement is required when handling a patient against his or her will.

1. All of the following are considered general medical complaints except:
   A. shortness of breath.
   B. headache.
   C. a twisted ankle.
   D. dizziness.

2. Reasons for a patient to have an altered level of consciousness include:
   A. poisoning.
   B. decreased levels of oxygen to the brain.
   C. head injury.
   D. all of the above.

3. The patient you are treating has a decrease in her level of responsiveness. This may be due to any of the following except:
   A. an injury to the lower (lumbar) spine.
   B. a psychiatric condition.
   C. hypoxia.
   D. low blood sugar.

4. When assessing and treating a patient with an altered mental status, the First Responder should:
   A. consider endotracheal intubation.
   B. determine the cause of the altered mental status.
   C. maintain an open airway.
   D. provide immediate defibrillation.

5. The first step in providing emergency medical care to a patient with an altered mental status is to do the:
   A. physical exam as needed.
   B. scene size-up.
   C. initial assessment.
   D. ongoing assessment.

6. When treating a patient with an altered mental status, of the following choices, your highest concern would be:
   A. listening for lung sounds.
   B. giving the patient sugar under the tongue.
   C. evaluating the need for airway adjuncts.
   D. none of the above.

7. The unresponsive nontraumatic patient should be placed in the _____ position and watched closely.
   A. face-down
   B. recovery
   C. shock
   D. head-up

8. A seizure may be caused by:
   A. low blood sugar level or hypoxia.
   B. brain tumors or head injury.
   C. complications of pregnancy or poisoning.
   D. all of the above.

9. Seizures usually last:
   A. less than 5 minutes.
   B. 5 to 10 minutes.
   C. 10 to 15 minutes.
   D. longer than 15 minutes.

10. The most serious complication that can occur during a seizure is:
    A. a brief period of unconsciousness.
    B. a laceration to the tongue.
    C. loss of bladder control.
    D. vomiting.

11. When caring for a seizure patient, the First Responder should:
    A. place a wallet in the corner of the patient's mouth.
    B. have a suction unit handy at the patient's side.
    C. restrain the patient to prevent movement.
    D. immobilize the back and neck right away.

12. If the seizure patient becomes bluish or cyanotic, the First Responder should:
    A. apply a non-rebreather mask.
    B. assist ventilations with a BVM and oxygen.
    C. insert a nasopharyngeal airway.
    D. none of the above.

13. When a patient is having a seizure that the First Responder witnesses, why is it important to describe to the EMT-Bs exactly what was seen?
    A. It will help convince them that you actually saw the seizure.

B. The patient will get taken care of faster.

C. The description could help determine the cause.

D. Some seizures are silent.

14. Patients who are more susceptible to cold injuries include:
    A. the very young.
    B. those experiencing alcohol or drug poisoning.
    C. the elderly.
    D. all of the above.

15. Which weather conditions contribute most to increased numbers of cold injuries?
    A. Light snow conditions
    B. Cold and dry
    C. Windy and damp
    D. Warm and rainy

16. Generalized cold exposure is called:
    A. heat stroke.
    B. hyperthermia.
    C. frostbite.
    D. hypothermia.

17. Patients with generalized cold exposure may have:
    A. stiff or rigid posture.
    B. shivering.
    C. muscular rigidity.
    D. all of the above.

18. Which of the following is not a sign or symptom of a generalized cold exposure?
    A. Frozen nose or fingertips
    B. Complaints of muscle stiffness
    C. Poor judgment about outer clothing
    D. Decreased mental status

19. The care of a hypothermia patient should include:
    A. covering wet clothing with warm blankets.
    B. assessing pulses for 30 to 45 seconds.
    C. quick handling of the patient.
    D. allowing the patient to have a cigarette to calm his or her nerves.

20. Body parts that often receive frostbite include the:
    A. ears.
    B. nose.
    C. toes.
    D. all of the above.

21. Another name for an early local cold injury is a _____ injury.
    A. frostbite
    B. superficial
    C. hypothermia
    D. deep

22. If a patient has a local cold injury with blisters evident, the First Responder should:
    A. wrap the patient with hot packs.
    B. never break the blisters.
    C. try to thaw out the body part.
    D. administer oxygen.

23. Often, a deep cold injury will present with:
    A. cold, yet soft skin.
    B. blanching of the skin.
    C. white, waxy skin.
    D. leaking blisters.

24. A superficial cold injury should not be:
    A. rubbed in snow.
    B. reexposed to the cold.
    C. massaged.
    D. all of the above.

25. Signs and symptoms of heat emergencies include:
    A. dizziness or faintness.
    B. rapid heart rate.
    C. weakness or exhaustion.
    D. all of the above.

26. Patients who are often susceptible to heat exposure include:
    A. the very old and the very young.
    B. athletes.
    C. people who live at high altitudes.
    D. all of the above.

27. The _____ the humidity, the _____ chance of a heat-related exposure.
    A. higher : greater
    B. higher : less
    C. lower : greater
    D. lower : less

28. When a person exercises he or she could lose as much as ____ of sweat per hour.
    A. 100 cc
    B. 500 cc
    C. 1 liter
    D. 3 liters

29. Treatment of the heat exposure emergency should include:
    A. rubbing the patient down with alcohol.
    B. dousing the patient in a pool of ice water.
    C. placing the patient in an air-conditioned environment.
    D having the patient drink plenty of water.

30. Abnormal behavior that is intolerable to others can be caused by:
    A. hypoglycemia.
    B. hypoxia.
    C. extremes of emotion.
    D. all of the above.

31. Examples of psychological crisis include:
    A. bizarre thinking or behavior.
    B. panic or agitation.
    C. self-destructive behavior.
    D. all of the above.

32. When assessing a behavioral emergency, the First Responder should:
    A. show that you are listening by rephrasing or repeating what is said.
    B. not tell the patient what you plan to do.
    C. be stern in your voice and tone.
    D. stare in the patient's eyes until you get their attention.

33. A precursor to violence may include the patient having:
    A. movement toward the First Responder.
    B. quick irregular movements.

C. clenched fists or a lethal object in hand.

D. all of the above.

34. When treating the patient with a behavioral emergency, the First Responder should:

A. tell the truth and not lie to the patient.

B. play along with any visual or auditory disturbances.

C. move swiftly and clear the scene as soon as possible.

D. stare him or her right in the eyes.

35. If a patient who has threatened suicide refuses to go to the hospital, the First Responder should:

A. consider involving medical command.

B. have him or her sign an RMA (refusal of medical aide).

C. restrain him or her immediately.

D. none of the above.

ANSWERS WITH RATIONALE

1. C. All of the following are considered general medical complaints: shortness of breath, headache, and dizziness. A twisted ankle is considered an injury.

2. D. Reasons for a patient to have an altered level of consciousness include: poisoning, decreased levels of oxygen to the brain (hypoxia), and head injury.

3. A. The patient you are treating has a decrease in her level of responsiveness. This may be due to any of the following: a psychiatric condition, hypoxia, or low blood sugar (hypoglycemia). The injury to the lower (lumbar) spine will probably not cause a decrease in the level of responsiveness.

4. C. When assessing and treating a patient with an altered mental status, the First Responder should maintain an open airway. Endotracheal intubation is an EMT-B optional skill or a skill of EMT-Intermediates or Paramedics. Defibrillation is not used unless the patient is in cardiac arrest and found in a shockable rhythm. It is not necessary to determine the cause of the altered mental status.

5. B. The first step in providing emergency medical care to a patient with an altered mental status is to do the scene size-up to assure that there is nothing that could harm the rescuers. The initial assessment, physical exam, and ongoing assessment may be conducted based on the patient's condition.

6. C. When treating a patient with an altered mental status, evaluating the need for airway adjuncts takes priority over listening for lung sounds or giving the patient sugar under the tongue for suspected hypoglycemia.

7. B. The unresponsive nontraumatic patient should be placed in the recovery position and watched closely. The face-down or (prone) position is rarely used in emergency care, due to the potential of complicating or closing off the airway. Both the head-up and shock positions would not allow secretions to drain out of the mouth on an unresponsive nontraumatic patient.

8. D. A seizure may be caused by low blood sugar level (hypoglycemia), low oxygen level (hypoxia), brain tumors, head injury, complications of pregnancy, or poisoning.

9. A. Seizures usually last for less than 5 minutes. If a seizure lasts for over 5 minutes, there may be some potential for brain damage, due to periods of hypoxia or anoxia (no oxygen at the cellular level).

10. D. A serious complication that can occur during a seizure is vomiting. This is serious because the patient could aspirate the foreign material into the lungs. It is not unusual for there to be a brief period of unconsciousness, laceration to the patient's tongue, or loss of bladder control.

11. B. When caring for a seizure patient, the First Responder should always have suction available at the patient's side, due to the potential of vomiting and secretions. Do not place a wallet in the corner of the patient's mouth or restrain the patient to prevent movement. Immobilization is not generally needed unless the seizure was due to a traumatic event. You may want to move the furniture so that the patient does not hurt himself or herself during the seizure.

12. B. If the seizure patient becomes bluish or cyanotic, the First Responder should assist ventilations with a BVM and oxygen. This is probably due to periods of apnea, which would not be corrected simply by putting in an NPA or non-rebreather mask alone.

13. C. When a patient is having a seizure that you witness, it important to describe to the EMT-Bs exactly what was seen so that they, in turn, can pass this important information on to the emergency department. The description can, in some instances, help with a diagnosis of the type of seizure and the location of the cause of the seizure in the brain.

14. D. Patients who are more susceptible to cold injuries include the very young, alcohol- or drug-poisoned patients, and the elderly.

15. C. Windy and damp weather conditions contribute the most to increased numbers of cold injuries. When dressing for outside, layer clothing to keep the cold wind out and to keep yourself dry.

16. D. Generalized cold exposure is called hypothermia. Heat stroke and hyperthermia are hot-weather injuries, and frostbite is a local cold-exposure injury.

17. D. Patients with generalized cold exposure may have a stiff or rigid posture, shivering, and muscular rigidity.

18. A. Signs or symptoms of a generalized cold exposure include complaints of muscle stiffness, poor judgment about outer clothing, and decreased mental status. A frozen nose or fingertips are signs of frostbite.

19. B. The care of a hypothermia patient should include assessing pulses for 30 to 45 seconds because the pulse rate is very slow. Do not cover wet clothing with warm blankets; rather, take off the wet clothing. Also beware that quick handling of a patient could cause ventricular fibrillation. Allowing the patient to have a cigarette dilates the vessels, making matters worse!

20. D. Common body parts for frostbite include the ears, nose, and toes.

21. B. Another name for an early local cold injury is a superficial injury. Frostbite is considered a late or deep cold injury. Hypothermia is a general cold injury.

22. B. If a patient has a local cold injury with blisters, the First Responder should never break the blisters. Wrapping a patient with hot packs may actually cause a burn or allow premature blood flow back into the frostbite area. Thawing out a frozen body part is recommended only if there is no chance that it could freeze again, so this is usually done in the hospital. Oxygen therapy is usually not necessary for frostbite unless there is a systemic problem.

23. C. Often, a deep cold injury will present with white, waxy skin. A superficial cold injury would present with skin that is cold, yet soft and blanching of the skin. Leaking blisters are not common.

24. D. A superficial cold injury should not be rubbed in snow, reexposed to the cold, or massaged.

25. D. Signs and symptoms of heat emergencies include dizziness or faintness, rapid heart rate, and weakness or exhaustion.

26. A. Patients who are often susceptible to heat exposure include the very old and the very young. Generally, athletes and people who live at high altitudes are attuned to environmental emergencies.

27. A. The higher the humidity, the greater the chance of a heat-related exposure. Humidity makes it difficulty for the body to get rid of heat through evaporation since there is already fluid in the air when it is high in humidity.

28. C. When exercising, a person can lose as much as 1 liter of sweat per hour.

29. C. Treatment of a heat exposure emergency should include placing the patient in an air-conditioned environment. Rubbing the patient down with alcohol is no longer recommended, as it is dangerous and could cause a fire! Dousing the patient in a pool of ice water is not needed; using wet towels at room temperature is adequate to bring down a patient's body temperature. Having a patient drink lots of fluids will only lead to a vomiting patient, since a patient in shock is probably not perfusing his or her digestive system adequately, making them more apt to vomit.

30. D. Abnormal behavior that is intolerable to others can be caused by hypoglycemia (low blood sugar), hypoxia (low oxygen in the blood), and extremes of emotion.

31. D. Examples of psychological crisis include bizarre thinking or behavior, panic or agitation, and self-destructive behavior.

32. A. When assessing a behavioral emergency, a First Responder should show that he or she is listening by rephrasing or repeating what is said. You will make the patient more paranoid by telling him or her what you plan to do. It is not necessary to be stern in your voice and tone. Staring at the patient will just make the person angry.

33. D. A precursor to violence may include the patient moving toward the First Responder, or exhibiting quick irregular movements, clenched fists, or a lethal object in the hand.

34. A. When treating a patient with a behavioral emergency, the First Responder tells the patient the truth. Do not play along with

visual or auditory disturbances. Moving swiftly and clearing the scene as soon as possible as well as stare him/her right in the eyes could cause the patient to become more aggitated.

35. A. If a patient who has threatened suicide refuses to go to the hospital, the First Responder should consider involving medical command. Do not let a patient threatening suicide sign an RMA. Restraining the patient would simply make matters worse.

LESSON **5-2** **Bleeding and Soft Tissues Injuries**

DOT OBJECTIVES

Cognitive Objectives

At the completion of this lesson, the First Responder student will be able to:

5-2.1 Differentiate between arterial, venous, and capillary bleeding.

5-2.2 State the emergency medical care for external bleeding.

5-2.3 Establish the relationship between body substance isolation and bleeding.

5-2.4 List the signs of internal bleeding.

5-2.5 List the steps in the emergency medical care of the patient with signs and symptoms of internal bleeding.

5-2.6 Establish the relationship between body substance isolation (BSI) and soft tissue injuries.

5-2.7 State the types of open soft tissue injuries.

5-2.8 Describe the emergency medical care of the patient with a soft tissue injury.

5-2.9 Discuss the emergency medical care considerations for a patient with a penetrating chest injury.

5-2.10 State the emergency medical care considerations for a patient with an open wound to the abdomen.

5-2.11 Describe the emergency medical care for an impaled object.

5-2.12 State the emergency medical care for an amputation.

5-2.13 Describe the emergency medical care for burns.

5-2.14 List the functions of dressing and bandaging.

Affective Objectives

At the completion of this lesson, the First Responder student will be able to:

5-2.15 Explain the rationale for body substance isolation when dealing with bleeding and soft tissue injuries.

5-2.16 Attend to the feelings of the patient with a soft tissue injury or bleeding.

5-2.17 Demonstrate a caring attitude towards patients with a soft tissue injury or bleeding who request emergency medical services.

5-2.18 Place the interests of the patient with a soft tissue injury or bleeding as the foremost consideration when making any and all patient care decisions.

5-2.19 Communicate with empathy to patients with a soft tissue injury or bleeding, as well as with family members and friends of the patient.

Psychomotor Objectives

At the completion of this lesson, the First Responder student will be able to:

5-2.20 Demonstrate direct pressure as a method of emergency medical care for external bleeding.

5-2.21 Demonstrate the use of diffuse pressure as a method of emergency medical care for external bleeding.

5-2.22 Demonstrate the use of pressure points as a method of emergency medical care for external bleeding.

5-2.23 Demonstrate the care of the patient exhibiting signs and symptoms of internal bleeding.

5-2.24 Demonstrate the steps in the emergency medical care of open soft tissue injuries.

5-2.25 Demonstrate the steps in the emergency medical care of a patient with an open chest wound.

5-2.26 Demonstrate the steps in the emergency medical care of a patient with open abdominal wounds.

5-2.27 Demonstrate the steps in the emergency medical care of a patient with an impaled object.

5-2.28 Demonstrate the steps in the emergency medical care of a patient with an amputation.

5-2.29 Demonstrate the steps in the emergency medical care of an amputated part.

QUICK REVIEW Bleeding may range from minor to life threatening. As a First Responder you may be called upon to control bleeding and care for many other types of soft tissue injuries. As you learned in Chapter 2, body substance isolation is designed to prevent contact between yourself and the infectious substances of another person. This is extremely important when controlling bleeding. Without the proper protective measures, you could be exposed to your patient's blood, exposing yourself to the risk of infectious disease.

When treating any patient, including those with the soft tissue injuries covered in this chapter, follow the patient assessment process. Begin with a thorough scene size-up. Be sure that the cause of the patient's soft tissue trauma will not harm you. Continue to the initial assessment, where you will treat life-threatening bleeding. The appropriate history and physical examination will follow. Patients with minor wounds will be treated after completing the assessment process, while patients with chest trauma or severe bleeding will be treated during the initial assessment. Patients who have open wounds will require calming and compassion, due to the visible nature of the wounds. Reassure the patient continually throughout the call.

Internal and External Bleeding

Bleeding is classified by the type of vessel from which the bleeding comes.

- *Arterial blood* is generally bright red and spurts from the wound. This is the most difficult bleeding to control.

- *Venous bleeding* flows steadily and does not spurt from the wound. The blood is darker red in color and may be profuse.

- *Capillary bleeding* oozes from the wound and the blood is also dark red in color. This type of bleeding may stop on its own.

Bleeding control is accomplished by the following methods:

1. *Fingertip pressure.* Apply pressure using the flat part of your gloved fingertips directly over the point of bleeding. Large wounds may require bulky dressings and the entire surface of your hand may be needed to apply pressure.

2. *Elevation.* If injuries are not suspected to the muscle or bone around the injury site, elevating the extremity may be used in conjunction with direct pressure.

3. *Hand pressure.* This type of pressure is used for large wounds, those that are too long or too wide to be controlled with fingertip pressure. Hand pressure may also be used when fingertip pressure fails to control the bleeding.

4. *Pressure points.* Pressure points are used in the extremities. The brachial pressure point is in the arm. To use the brachial pressure point, use firm fingertip pressure approximately halfway down the humerus. The pressure point is obtained by compressing the brachial artery against the humerus. The pulse is felt between the muscle and the bone and may require considerable pressure, depending on the patient's size. The femoral pressure point is used for bleeding in the leg. This pressure point is found near the crease formed between the upper thigh and the groin. Pressure is applied with the heel of a hand directly over where the pulse is felt. It is important to know the location of these pressure points because they are also used to locate pulses in pediatric patients.

Internal bleeding is caused by injured or damaged internal structures. This can lead to extensive bleeding that is hidden under the skin. The signs and symptoms of internal bleeding include increased pulse and respiratory rate, skin which is cool and pale, nausea and vomiting, thirst, and mental status changes. (These are the signs and symptoms of shock, which is discussed later in the chapter.) There may be pain, discoloration, hardening, or swelling of the tissues involved in the bleeding. If trauma is involved, examine the mechanism of injury to determine the possibility of internal bleeding. Even musculoskeletal injuries such as a fractured femur may cause serious internal bleeding.

Caring for a patient who has suspected internal bleeding or a mechanism of injury that could cause internal bleeding is as follows:

1. Complete the patient assessment process, including the size-up, initial assessment, physical examination, and ongoing exams. Reassure the patient continuously throughout the call.

2. Take body substance isolation precautions.

3. Maintain the airway. Ventilate if necessary.

4. Manage any external bleeding.

5. If there are no spinal injuries, place the patient in a position of comfort. Keep the patient warm.

6. Treat for shock.

Shock

Shock is also known as *hypoperfusion*. This is an abnormal condition resulting from inadequate delivery of oxygenated blood to body tissues. It may be caused by many factors, including loss of blood or the heart's inability to circulate oxygenated blood.

The signs and symptoms of shock are:

- Thirst

- Restlessness, anxiety

- Rapid, weak pulse

- Rapid, shallow respirations

- Mental status changes

- Pale, cool, moist skin

When you encounter a patient with significant traumatic injury, you will suspect and treat for shock. Complete the patient assessment process and follow the following treatment steps:

1. Maintain the airway and provide ventilation if required.

2. Prevent further blood loss.

3. Keep the patient calm and in a position of comfort. If the patient has spinal injuries, maintain stabilization of the neck and spine.

4. Do not give the patient anything to eat or drink.

5. Provide care for specific injuries as outlined in this and other chapters.

Wounds and Injuries

Wounds may be classified as open or closed, by severity, and by location on the body. There are three basic types of open wounds:

1. *Abrasions.* Commonly referred to as *scrapes*, these wounds result when the skin comes in forceful contact with a harsh surface. These injuries generally bleed very little but can be extremely painful.

2. *Lacerations.* Lacerations are a break in the skin. These may be smooth or jagged and of varying depths. Lacerations may be caused by a sharp object, such as a knife, and bleeding could be severe.

3. *Penetrating or puncture wounds.* These wounds are caused by sharp objects or projectiles that are fired at the body. In the case of penetrating wounds, there may be an exit as well as an entrance wound. Because the item or projectile penetrates the skin, the amount of damage is difficult to estimate. There may be slight external bleeding but severe internal bleeding. Examples of these wounds would be caused by knives or bullets.

When you encounter a soft tissue injury, perform a complete patient assessment. Body substance isolation is important in these cases. Your care for the patient with a soft tissue injury is:

1. Expose the wound.

2. Control bleeding.

3. Prevent contamination.

4. Apply a sterile dressing to the wound and bandage it in place.

There are several soft tissue injuries that extend to the underlying tissues. There are special considerations when you treat these patients.

1. *Chest injuries.* When there is an open wound to the chest or back, an occlusive dressing must be applied over the wound.

This is because air entering the chest cavity will disrupt the critical pressures required to breathe. The dressing must be occlusive, such as foil or thick plastic wrap. Tape three sides of this dressing in place. Monitor the airway and be prepared to assist ventilations if necessary.

2. *Impaled Objects.* Impaled objects are foreign objects that have penetrated the skin and remain in place. You must not remove impaled objects unless they interfere with CPR, airway control, or are in the cheek. Manually secure the object in place using bulky dressings and control bleeding around the object.

3. *Eviscerations.* Eviscerations are open injuries with protruding organs. This is most commonly seen around the abdomen. Cover the organs with saline-moistened dressings. Never replace an organ that is protruding from the body.

4. *Amputations.* When a part of the body is severed or amputated, place the part in a plastic bag. Place the bag containing the body part in a larger container with ice and water. Do not submerge the part directly in water or allow the part to freeze. Do not use dry ice. Control bleeding as necessary.

Burns

Burns may be caused by heat, flame, chemicals, or electricity. Burns are classified according to depth. Superficial burns involve reddening of the outer layers of skin. Partial thickness burns involve the outer and middle layers of skin. These burns are red, painful, and have blisters. Full-thickness burns extend through all layers of skin. There will be charring of the skin along with redness and blisters.

Complete a patient assessment. Remember that there may be airway problems associated with burns around the face or when heated air was inhaled in a closed space. When caring for a burn patient:

1. Stop the burning process with water or saline.

2. Monitor the airway carefully.

3. Prevent further contamination.

4. Cover the burned areas with a dry, sterile dressing.

5. Never use ointments or lotions. Do not break blisters.

Burns that are caused by chemicals pose specific problems. Protect yourself from contamination. If the chemical is a powder, brush it off before irrigating the area. Make sure that the dry chemical does not react with water. When irrigating a chemical burn use large quantities of water for at least 15 minutes.

Electrical burns also require special attention to scene safety. These burns may also cause a condition more serious than that which would appear from the surface. Electricity passing through the body can cause unseen tissue damage and alter the conduction of the heart, leading to cardiac or respiratory arrest.

Infants and children have a greater body surface area in relation to their total body size and therefore lose more heat and fluids when burned. The environment in which the child is treated must be kept warm to prevent heat loss.

Dressing and Bandaging

Dressings are usually sterile and are meant to go directly on the wound. The dressings are used to stop bleeding, to protect the area from further damage, and to prevent contamination. Examples of dressings are 4 x 4 gauze pads, combination dressings, and occlusive dressings.

Bandages hold the dressing in place. They do not have direct contact with the wound and need not be sterile. Examples of bandages are roller gauze, triangular bandages, and tape.

REVIEW QUESTIONS

1. Arterial bleeding is characterized by which of the following?
   A. Dark red, steadily flowing blood
   B. Bright red, spurting blood
   C. Dark red, slowly oozing blood
   D. Can occur only in the chest area

2. Capillary bleeding is characterized by which of the following?
   A. Dark red, steadily flowing blood
   B. Bright red, spurting blood
   C. Dark red, slowly oozing blood
   D. Can occur only in the chest area

3. Which of the following statements about treating a bleeding patient is false?
   A. Bleeding patients should be calmed and reassured.
   B. Direct pressure is used for bleeding control.

C. Pressure points may be used to control abdominal bleeding.

D. Body substance isolation is important while controlling bleeding.

4. The steps for bleeding control, in order, are:
   A. fingertip pressure, elevation, hand pressure, pressure point.
   B. pressure point, elevation, fingertip pressure.
   C. hand pressure, elevation, pressure point, fingertip pressure.
   D. pressure point, pressure, elevation.

5. A patient who has uncontrolled arterial bleeding would cause you to wear which of the following pieces of personal protective equipment?
   A. Gloves
   B. Mask and eye protection
   C. Gown
   D. All of the above

6. The brachial pressure point is located in the:
   A. rib.
   B. hip.
   C. neck.
   D. arm.

7. A pressure point compresses:
   A. a muscle against a bone.
   B. an artery against a bone.
   C. an artery against a muscle.
   D. none of the above.

8. Which of the following statements about bleeding control is false?
   A. The scene size-up may be skipped if the patient is bleeding severely.
   B. Body substance isolation must be used when controlling bleeding.
   C. The patient will require calming and reassurance during your care.
   D. Elevation should not be used if there is an injury to the muscle or bone.

9. Which of the following statements about internal bleeding is true?
   A. Internal bleeding is usually not serious.
   B. Injuries to bones may cause internal bleeding.
   C. A laceration is a type of internal bleeding.
   D. Fingertip pressure is recommended to control internal bleeding.

10. Which of the following signs or symptoms of internal bleeding is false?
    A. Pale, cool skin
    B. Thirst
    C. Nausea and vomiting
    D. Decreased pulse and respiratory rate

11. Internal injury may be identified by which of the following?
    A. Mechanism of injury
    B. Discolored tissue
    C. Swollen or hard tissue
    D. All of the above

12. The difference between a dressing and a bandage is:
    A. bandages are sterile and go directly over a wound.
    B. dressings are used to hold bandages in place.
    C. bandages are used to hold dressings in place.
    D. bandages are sterile, dressings are not.

13. Shock is best defined as:
    A. uncontrolled bleeding.
    B. failure of the body to deliver oxygenated blood to body tissues.
    C. abnormal constriction of the blood vessels throughout the body.
    D. heart failure.

14. Shock is also called:
    A. cardiac syndrome.
    B. traumatic asphyxia.
    C. hypoperfusion.
    D. hypoglycemia.

15. An abrasion is best described as:
    A. a deep wound with steady bleeding.
    B. a painful injury to the outermost layers of skin with heavy bleeding.

C. a painful injury to the outermost layers of skin with very little bleeding.

D. a wound usually caused by a knife or gunshot.

16. A laceration is best described as any wound:
    A. caused by a sharp object, which may bleed severely.
    B. caused by a scraping motion.
    C. with an object remaining in the patient.
    D. with minor bleeding.

17. Which of the following statements about penetrating and puncture wounds is false?
    A. These injuries may leave entrance and exit wounds.
    B. There may be little or no external bleeding.
    C. The internal bleeding is always minor with such wounds.
    D. These wounds are caused by a projectile or sharp object.

18. An open wound to the chest is best treated by which of the following methods?
    A. Direct pressure and elevation
    B. Application of an occlusive dressing sealed on three sides
    C. Application of an occlusive dressing sealed on four sides
    D. Omitting a dressing to the chest because the lung may collapse.

19. In which of the following conditions would it be acceptable to remove an impaled object?
    A. For an object impaled in the cheek
    B. For an object that interferes with chest compressions
    C. For an object that interferes with airway management
    D. All of the above

20. An evisceration is:
    A. A wound where a body part has been torn from the body.
    B. An extremity injury with regular edges.
    C. A type of closed head injury.
    D. A wound with organs protruding.

21. Which of the following treatments would not be appropriate when caring for an amputated body part?
    A. Place the part in a plastic bag, then place that bag in a larger bag with ice and water.
    B. Do not allow the amputated part to freeze.

C. Place the amputated part on dry ice.

D. Control bleeding from the injury site as required.

22. Charred skin is a characteristic of which classification of burn?
    A. Superficial
    B. Partial-thickness
    C. Full-thickness
    D. Fourth-degree

23. Reddening of the skin alone is characteristic of which classification of burn?
    A. Superficial
    B. Partial-thickness
    C. Full-thickness
    D. Fourth-degree

24. Reddening of the skin with blisters and severe pain are characteristics of which classification of burn?
    A. Superficial
    B. Partial-thickness
    C. Full-thickness
    D. Multidermal

25. Which of the following treatments is appropriate for a patient with a burn injury?
    A. Breaking blisters
    B. Using ointment on full-thickness burns
    C. Covering the burn with a dry, sterile dressing
    D. All of the above

26. When treating a patient with a chemical burn involving dry powder:
    A. flush the area immediately with large quantities of water.
    B. brush the powder off before flushing with water.
    C. do not transport because powders cannot burn.
    D. none of the above.

27. Which of the following statements regarding burns in infants and children is false?
    A. Children have greater surface area in relation to total body size than that of adults.
    B. Children have less surface area in relation to total body size than that of adults.

C. Children may have greater heat and fluid loss than that of adults when burned.

D. Burns may be the result of child abuse.

28. Electrical burns:

A. are often more severe than they appear on the surface.

B. may cause respiratory or cardiac arrest.

C. require attention to scene safety.

D. all of the above.

29. Burns should be covered with:

A. a dry, sterile dressing.

B. a moist, sterile dressing.

C. ointment, then a dressing.

D. isopropyl alcohol–soaked dressing.

30. Emergency care for burns includes:

A. monitoring the patient for airway problems and closure.

B. stopping the burning process.

C. removing smoldering clothing and jewelry.

D. all of the above.

ANSWERS WITH RATIONALE

1. B. Arterial bleeding is characterized by bright red, spurting blood. This is because arterial blood is under the greatest pressure, having just left the heart. The other types of bleeding are discussed in subsequent answers.

2. C. Capillary bleeding comes from the smallest type of blood vessels. It is dark red and oozing. Venous blood is also dark red but flows faster than capillary bleeding.

3. C. Pressure points are used for extremities and not for abdominal bleeding. The brachial pressure point is used to control bleeding in the arm. The femoral pressure point is used to control bleeding in the leg.

4. A. If you were trained in a prior curriculum or first-aid class, you may notice a slight difference here. Direct pressure is broken down into two parts: fingertip pressure and direct hand pressure. Fingertip pressure is used first, especially on smaller wounds. This provides more intense pressure directly over the wound. If the wound is within an uninjured extremity, it may be elevated. If this

does not control the bleeding, pressure using the entire hand may be required. This hand pressure is also indicated for larger wounds. Use of pressure points is the final step to control bleeding.

5. D. Arterial bleeding is spurting and abundant. This requires that First Responders use gloves, mask and eye protection, and a gown.

6. D. The brachial pressure point is located in the midshaft humerus, the upper arm.

7. B. A pressure point controls bleeding by compressing an artery against a bone.

8. A. The scene size-up may never be skipped. This is where you ensure your own safety. If you do not remain safe, you will not be able to control bleeding or perform other emergency care procedures.

9. B. Injuries to bones will cause internal bleeding. A fracture to the femur can cause up to 1 liter of blood loss. Internal bleeding is usually serious and is not controlled by fingertip pressure. A laceration is an external injury.

10. D. Shock will cause an *increased* pulse and respiratory rate, not a decreased rate as choice D states. The other signs and symptoms listed are correct.

11. D. All the choices listed are indications of internal bleeding. Discolored and swollen hard tissue is a result of blood accumulation beneath the skin and other responses of the body to the internal bleeding. The mechanism of injury is important because it indicates that internal injuries are *possible*. This is will help in identifying shock very early in your care.

12. C. Dressings should be sterile because they contact the wound directly. Bandages hold dressings in place. Since bandages do not come directly in contact with the wound, they need not be sterile.

13. B. Shock is defined as the inability of the body to deliver oxygenated blood to the organs and tissues of the body. Frequently, this is due to reduced blood volume, as seen in severe or internal bleeding. Uncontrolled bleeding and heart failure may be causes of shock, but they are not definitions. The body tries to compensate for blood loss by constricting blood vessels during shock.

14. C. Shock is also called hypoperfusion. *Hypo* indicates "under." As you will recall from the preceding question, shock

means that there is reduced blood flow to the body's tissues. The tissues are therefore underperfused or hypoperfused.

15. C. An abrasion, commonly referred to as a scrape, is painful but results in very little bleeding. Abrasions affect the outermost layers of skin.

16. A. A laceration is a wound caused by a sharp object such as a knife. Lacerations may be of varying depths and may bleed severely. Scraping motions generally result in abrasions. When an object remains in the patient, it is referred to as impaled. Choice D is not specific enough to classify as a particular wound.

17. C. The internal bleeding that occurs with penetrating and puncture wounds has the potential to affect internal organs and be quite severe. These types of wounds may involve both entrance and exit areas (as in a gunshot wound), may not bleed severely on the outside, and are caused by projectiles and sharp objects.

18. B. An occlusive dressing to seal the wound is an important part of caring for a patient with an open wound to the chest. The dressing should be sealed on *three* sides so that air will be prevented from entering the chest cavity but will be allowed to leave. Remember that injuries over a patient's back also affect the chest cavity.

19. D. Impaled objects may be removed in all the situations listed. The reason that an impaled object is often left in place is that its removal may cause additional internal injury. It is difficult to tell if the path through which the object is to be removed is the path by which it went in. Impaled objects in the cheek are an exception since you are able to reach both sides of the object. When an object interferes with airway management or chest compression, when needed, the object must be removed.

20. D. An evisceration is a wound with organs protruding and is most frequently thought of as a wound to the abdomen where intestines protrude.

21. C. Dry ice should never be used when caring for an amputated part. It is correct to place the amputated part in a bag, then place that bag in another bag which contains ice or water. Never submerge an amputated part in water, place it in direct contact with ice, or allow it to freeze.

22. C. Charred skin is characteristic of full-thickness burns. These are the most severe. Superficial is the least severe, followed by partial-thickness, with full-thickness being the most severe.

23. A. Reddening of the skin in the least severe sign of burn and is seen in superficial burns. The classification system refers to depth of the burn.

24. B. The burn described in this question is a partial-thickness burn. Full-thickness burns involve charring, while superficial burns are characterized by reddening of the upper layers of skin.

25. C. Covering a burn with a dry, sterile dressing is appropriate care. Do not break blisters or apply ointments in the field.

26. B. Dry powders should be brushed off before applying water. There are dry powders that may react with water and cause much greater damage to the skin wet than dry. After the powder has been brushed away, it is appropriate to flush the area with large quantities of water.

27. B. Children have a greater surface area in relation to total body size. Choice B is false because it states that children have a *smaller* surface area. This is important because the greater surface area can result in greater heat and fluid loss.

28. D. All the statements listed are true about electrical burns. They travel through the body and may cause entrance *and* exit wounds. The electrical shock may interrupt the electrical rhythm of the heart, causing cardiac arrest. Scene safety is important to prevent accidental shock and injury to EMS personnel.

29. A. Burns should be covered with a dry, sterile dressing. Avoid the use of ointments or other substances. Moist dressings are not recommended in the curriculum, but this may vary in local protocols.

30. D. The care for burns includes all the choices in this question. It is important to monitor the patient for airway problems. Superheated air may cause airway narrowing or closure. Some patients may still be on fire or quite hot. Always stop the burning process. Smoldering clothing and jewelry may be removed if not melted into or stuck to the burn.

LESSON 5-3 Injuries to Muscles and Bones

DOT OBJECTIVES

Cognitive Objectives

At the completion of this lesson, the First Responder student will be able to:

5-3.1   Describe the function of the musculoskeletal system.

5-3.2   Differentiate between an open and a closed painful, swollen, deformed extremity.

5-3.3   List the emergency medical care for a patient with a painful, swollen, deformed extremity.

5-3.4   Relate mechanism of injury to potential injuries of the head and spine.

5-3.5   State the signs and symptoms of a potential spine injury.

5-3.6   Describe the method of determining if a responsive patient may have a spine injury.

5-3.7   List the signs and symptoms of injury to the head.

5-3.8   Describe the emergency medical care for injuries to the head.

Affective Objectives

At the completion of this lesson, the First Responder student will be able to:

5-3.9 Explain the rationale for immobilization of the painful, swollen, deformed extremity.

5-3.10 Demonstrate a caring attitude towards patients with a musculoskeletal injury who request emergency medical services.

5-3.11 Place the interests of the patient with a musculoskeletal injury as the foremost consideration when making any and all patient care decisions.

5-3.12 Communicate with empathy to patients with a musculoskeletal injury, as well as with family members and friends of the patient.

Psychomotor Objectives

At the completion of this lesson, the First Responder student will be able to:

5-3.13 Demonstrate the emergency medical care of a patient with a painful, swollen, deformed extremity.

5-3.14 Demonstrate opening the airway in a patient with suspected spinal cord injury.

5-3.15 Demonstrate evaluating a responsive patient with a suspected spinal cord injury.

5-3.16 Demonstrate stabilizing of the cervical spine.

QUICK REVIEW

Extremity Injuries

The function of the skeletal system is to give the body shape and protect the vital organs. Any break in the continuity of the skin associated with a *painful, swollen, deformed extremity* is classified as an *open musculoskeletal injury*. If there is no break in the skin, it is classified as a *closed injury*.

The signs and symptoms of a painful, swollen, deformed extremity (PSDE) include:

- Deformity or angulation
- Pain and tenderness

- Grating

- Swelling

- Bruising or discoloration

- Exposed bone ends

- Joints locked into position

The emergency medical care for a patient with a painful, swollen, deformed extremity includes:

1. Assure body substance isolation.

2. After life threats have been controlled, allow the patient to remain in a position of comfort.

3. Apply a cold pack to the area of the PSDE to reduce swelling and pain.

4. Manual extremity stabilization, involving:
   a. Support the injury above and below.
   b. Cover open wounds with a sterile dressing.
   c. Use a pad to prevent pressure and discomfort to the patient.
   d. When in doubt, manually stabilize the injury.
   e. Do not intentionally replace protruding bones.

Head and Spine Injuries

Injuries to the head and spine can be devastating. The mechanisms of injury that most often involve head and spine injuries include the following:

- Motor vehicle vs. motor vehicle crashes

- Pedestrian vs. vehicle crashes

- Falls

- Blunt trauma

- Penetrating trauma to the head, neck, or torso

- Motorcycle crashes

- Springboard or platform diving accidents

- Unresponsive trauma patients

The signs and symptoms of a potential spine injury include any or all of the following:

- Tenderness at the injury site

- Pain upon moving (it is important not to "test" for pain by encouraging the patient to move, as this could cause serious injury)

- Pain not associated with movement or palpation along the spinal column or lower legs, which can be constant or intermittent

- Soft tissue injuries associated with trauma to the head, neck or cervical spine, shoulders, back or abdomen, thoracic or lumbar, and/or lower extremities

- Numbness, weakness, or tingling in the extremities

- Loss of sensation or paralysis below the suspected level of injury

- Loss of sensation or paralysis in the upper extremities

- Respiratory impairment

- Loss of bladder and/or bowel control

- Ability of the patient to work, move extremities, or feel sensation (note that a lack of pain to the spinal column does not rule out the possibility of spinal column or cord damage)

When assessing the responsive patient for a possible spine injury, the First Responder should consider the mechanism of injury as well as asking the patient a series of questions, such as:

- Does your neck or back hurt?

- What happened?

- Where does it hurt?

- Can you move your hands and feet?

- Can you feel me touching your fingers?

- Can you feel me touching your toes?

If the patient is unresponsive, the First Responder will need to maintain airway and breathing while stabilizing the head and neck manually in the position in which it was found or in a neutral position while trying to determine the mechanism of injury.

Injuries to the brain and skull may be open or closed. Open injuries may present with bleeding, while closed injuries may present with swelling or depression of skull bones. Injuries to the scalp may bleed more than expected due to the large number of blood vessels in the scalp. An actual injury to the brain tissue or bleeding inside the skull may increase pressure [intracranial pressure or (ICP)] on the brain due to swelling within the skull (cranium).

The emergency medical care for a patient with a suspected head injury includes:

1. Provide body substance isolation.

2. Maintain airway/artificial ventilation and oxygenation.

3. Do the initial assessment with manual spinal stabilization on the scene.

4. Monitor the mental status of the patient closely for possible deterioration.

5. Control bleeding by applying enough pressure to control the bleeding, without disturbing the underlying tissue. Be sure to dress and bandage open wounds.

6. Be prepared for changes in patient conditions.

To summarize, a patient who has a potential musculoskeletal injury and exhibits a painful, swollen, deformed extremity or injury to the head or spine should be immobilized until the time when they can be medically cleared by a higher-trained medical professional, probably with the aid of an x-ray. Since musculoskeletal injuries can prove to be very disabling, the First Responder must always provide a caring attitude toward patients, as they are apt to be very scared.

REVIEW QUESTIONS

1. The function of the musculoskeletal system includes all of the following except:
   A. protecting the vital organs.
   B. developing the hormone insulin.

C. giving the body its shape.

D. none of the above.

2. Why is it important to differentiate between an open and a closed painful, swollen, deformed extremity?

A. Because an open PSDE may require bleeding control

B. Because a closed PSDE involves no bleeding

C. Because the closed PSDE will be more painful

D. Because the open PSDE need not be immobilized

3. When treating a PSDE:

A. provide manual extremity stabilization.

B. cover open wounds with a sterile dressing.

C. apply cold to reduce swelling.

D. all of the above.

4. Of the following, which is not a common mechanism of injury for both head injury and spine injury?

A. Motor vehicle collisions

B. Springboard or platform diving accidents

C. Falls from heights

D. Hangings

5. Treatment of a PSDE should include all of the following except:

A. support above and below the injury.

B. application of a pressure bandage to all exposed bone ends.

C. avoiding intentional replacement of protruding bone ends.

D. manual stabilization of the injury.

6. Signs and symptoms of a potential spine injury include all of the following except:

A. tenderness at the injury site.

B. a burning sensation in the abdomen.

C. loss of sensation above the suspected injury site.

D. numbness in the extremities.

7. If the patient is unresponsive after falling from a roof onto his or her back, the First Responder should first:

A. maintain airway and breathing while stabilizing the head and neck.

B. splint any leg injuries as soon as possible.

C. determine the distance from the ground.

D. all of the above.

8. Immobilization of a spine injury should continue until:

A. the patient begins to move the legs.

B. sensation returns in the legs.

C. the patient is cleared by an EMT-B.

D. none of the above.

9. Injuries to the scalp:

A. do not involve arterial bleeding.

B. may bleed more than expected.

C. do not bleed freely.

D. do not involve venous bleeding.

10. The emergency medical care of a head-injured patient involves:

A. initial assessment on the scene.

B. maintaining oxygenation, if trained to do so.

C. body substance isolation.

D. all of the above.

11. When an 18-year-old female strikes a tree with her head while skiing, you should initially assist the patient by:

A. providing an initial assessment with manual spinal stabilization.

B. helping her get up to walk it off.

C. controlling bleeding with a pressure bandage.

D. all of the above.

12. Care of a head-injured patient should include:

A. transport in the shock position.

B. rapid rewarming of the injury.

C. close monitoring of mental status.

D. none of the above.

13. An actual injury to the brain may _____ pressure on the brain.

A. eliminate

B. increase

C. decrease

D. double

14. When assessing a responsive patient for a possible spine injury, the First Responder should ask the patient:

A. if he or she can move his or her toes.

B. if his or her back hurts.

C. if he or she can feel his or her fingers.

D. all of the above.

15. The assessment of a musculoskeletal injury should always include:

A. splinting and transport.

B. distal pulse, motor, and sensation checks.

C. full range-of-motion checks.

D. none of the above.

ANSWERS WITH RATIONALE

1. B. The function of the musculoskeletal system includes protecting the vital organs and giving the body its shape. It does not include development of the hormone insulin, which is manufactured in the pancreas.

2. A. It is important to differentiate between an open and a closed painful, swollen, deformed extremity because an open PSDE can require bleeding control.

3. D. When treating a PSDE, provide manual extremity stabilization, cover open wounds with a sterile dressing, and apply cold to reduce swelling.

4. D. Hanging is not a common mechanism of injury for both head injury and spine injury, whereas motor vehicle collisions, springboard or platform diving accidents, and falls from heights are.

5. B. The treatment of a PSDE should include support above and below the injury, not intentionally replacing protruding bone ends, and manual stabilization of the injury. Do not apply a pressure bandage to exposed bone ends.

6. C. Signs and symptoms of a potential spine injury include tenderness at the injury site, a burning sensation in the abdomen, and numbness in the extremities. An injury to the spine may cause loss of sensation below the suspected injury site, not above.

7. A. If the patient is unresponsive after falling from a roof onto his or her back, the First Responder should maintain airway and

breathing while stabilizing the head and neck. Splinting any leg injuries as soon as possible or determining the distance from the ground are not immediate priorities.

8. D. Immobilization of a spine injury should continue until the patient is cleared by a higher medical authority, such as a physician in the emergency department. The return of sensation suggests nerve sensation, not repair to broken bones.

9. B. Injuries to the scalp may bleed more than expected. They can involve arterial or venous as well as capillary bleeding.

10. D. The emergency medical care of a head-injured patient involves initial assessment on the scene, maintaining oxygenation (if trained to do so), and body substance isolation.

11. A. When an 18-year-old female strikes a tree with her head while skiing, you should initially assist the patient by providing an initial assessment with manual spinal stabilization. Do not help her get up to walk it off. A pressure bandage is not generally used on a head injury.

12. C. Care of the head-injured patient should include close monitoring of mental status since the earliest signs of a head-injured patient's condition are often subtle changes in mental status. These patients are either transported in the head-up position or immobilized to a spineboard. Rapid rewarming is not appropriate for this type of injury.

13. B. An actual injury to the brain may increase pressure on the brain. This is due to the limited room for expansion within the cranium when the contused brain tries to swell.

14. D. When assessing a responsive patient for a possible spine injury the First Responder should ask the patient if he or she can move his or her toes, if his or her back hurts, and if he or she can feel his or her fingers.

15. B. The assessment of a musculoskeletal injury should always include distal pulse, motor, and sensation checks. Full range-of-motion checks are not done in the field prior to an x-ray, and splinting and transport are not considered assessment steps.

6-1 Childbirth

**D O T
OBJECTIVES**

Cognitive Objectives

At the completion of this lesson, the First Responder student will be able to:

6-1.1 Identify the following structures: birth canal, placenta, umbilical cord, amniotic sac.

6-1.2 Define the following terms: crowning, bloody show, labor, abortion.

6-1.3 State the indications of an imminent delivery.

6-1.4 State the steps in the pre-delivery preparation of the mother.

6-1.5 Establish the relationship between body substance isolation and childbirth.

6-1.6 State the steps to assist in the delivery.

6-1.7 Describe care of the baby as the head appears.

6-1.8 Discuss the steps in the delivery of the placenta.

6-1.9 List the steps in the emergency medical care of the mother post-delivery.

6-1.10 Discuss the steps in caring for a newborn.

Affective Objectives

At the completion of this lesson, the First Responder student will be able to:

6-1.11 Explain the rationale for attending to the feeling of a patient in need of emergency medical care during childbirth.

6-1.12 Demonstrate a caring attitude towards patients during childbirth who request emergency medical services.

6-1.13 Place the interests of the patient during childbirth as the foremost consideration when making any and all patient care decisions.

6-1.14 Communicate with empathy to patients during childbirth, as well as with family members and friends of the patient.

Psychomotor Objectives

At the completion of this lesson, the First Responder student will be able to:

6-1.15 Demonstrate the steps to assist in the normal cephalic delivery.

6-1.16 Demonstrate necessary care procedures of the fetus as the head appears.

6-1.17 Attend to the steps in the delivery of the placenta.

6-1.18 Demonstrate the post-delivery care of the mother.

6-1.19 Demonstrate the care of the newborn.

QUICK REVIEW There are a number of terms to learn in this lesson. The First Responder should be able to define these terms: birth canal, placenta. umbilical cord, amniotic sac, crowning, bloody show, and abortion. The *birth canal* consists of the vagina and the lower part of the uterus. The *placenta* is the organ through which the fetus exchanges nourishment and waste products during pregnancy. The *umbilical cord* is an extension of the placenta through which the fetus receives nourishment while in the uterus. The *amniotic sac* is commonly called the bag of waters. It is the sac that surrounds the fetus inside the uterus. *Crowning* is the bulging out of the vagina, which is opening as the fetus's head or presenting part presses against it. A *bloody show* occurs when mucus and blood exit the vagina as labor begins. The muscular contractions of the uterus beginning with the first uterine contraction and ending with the delivery of the placenta is called *labor*. An *abortion*, often called a miscarriage by nonmedical personnel, is the delivery of the products of conception early in the pregnancy.

To determine if delivery is imminent, the First Responder should ask the patient: What is your due date? Any chance of multiple births? Any bleeding or discharge? Does the patient feel as if she is having a bowel movement with increasing pressure in the vaginal area? If the patient answers yes to the preceding questions, examine for crowning. If crowning is present, the First Responder should prepare for a prehospital delivery. Don your body substance isolation equipment. This includes eye protection, mouth protection, disposable gloves, and because of the potential for blood splattering, a gown to keep your uniform clean. Childbirth in the field is not common. It does, however, give a high potential of exposure to body substances during delivery if you are not properly protected.

The First Responder should not touch the vaginal areas except during delivery and with a partner present. Do not let the mother go to the bathroom, as the urge to move her bowels is usually from pressure caused by an infant in the birth canal. Do not hold the mother's legs together in an attempt to hold back or delay the delivery.

The procedure the First Responder should take to assist in the delivery should first be body substances isolation. Have the mother lie on her back with her knees drawn up and legs spread apart. Place absorbent, clean materials under the patient's buttocks and elevate her buttocks with a blanket or pillow.

When the infant's head appears, place the palm of your hand on top of the delivering baby's head, exerting very gentle pressure to prevent an explosive delivery. If the amniotic sac does not break or has not broken, tear it with your fingers and push it away from the infant's head and mouth. As the infant's head is being born, determine if the umbilical cord is wrapped around the infant's neck. If it is, attempt to slip the cord over the infant's head and shoulders. If this is not successful, attempt to alleviate pressure on the cord.

After the infant's head is born, support the head. Next suction the mouth and then the nostrils two or three times with a bulb syringe. Use caution to avoid contact with the back of the infant's mouth. If a bulb syringe is not available, wipe the infant's mouth and then the nose with gauze.

As the torso and full body are born, support the infant with both hands. Do not pull on the infant. As the feet are delivered, grasp the feet. Keep the infant level with the mother's vagina. You may place the infant on the mother's abdomen for warmth. When the umbilical cord stops pulsating, it should be tied with gauze between the mother and the infant so you can place the infant on the mother's abdomen.

Wipe blood and mucus from the infant's mouth and nose with sterile gauze, suction the mouth and then nose again, and then dry the infant. Try rubbing the baby's back or flicking the soles of its feet to stimulate breathing. First Responders should never hold a newborn upside down by the legs. This may be done on television, but in the real world the infant would be too slippery and you might drop him or her!

Wrap the infant in a warm blanket and place the infant on its side with the head slightly lower than the trunk. There is no need to cut the cord in a normal delivery. However, your local medical director may be opinionated on this issue and chose to train you how to cut the cord properly. Be sure to record the time of delivery.

If there is a chance of multiple births, prepare for the second delivery. Next observe for delivery of the placenta. This may take up to 30 minutes. If the placenta is delivered, wrap it in a towel with three-fourths of the umbilical cord and place in a plastic bag, keeping the bag at the level of the infant. Place a sterile pad over the vaginal opening, lower the mother's legs and help her hold them together.

The mother will have vaginal bleeding following the delivery. Up to 300 to 500 mL of blood loss is well tolerated by a mother following delivery. The First Responder must be aware of this loss so as not to cause undue psychological stress on himself or herself or the new mother. With continued blood loss the First Responder should massage the uterus by using the hand with the fingers fully extended, placing the palms on the lower abdomen above the pubis. Massage by kneading over the area. If bleeding continues, check your massage technique. Another way to help contract the uterus to slow the bleeding is to allow the mother to nurse the infant. This will release a hormone in the mother that causes her uterus to constrict.

Initial care of the newborn involves assessment of the pulse and respiratory status. The pulse should be greater than 100 per minute. You can take the pulse at the umbilical cord or the brachial artery. The respiratory status should show a rate of 40 or more and a child who can cry. The most important care that the First Responder can provide is to position, dry, keep warm, and stimulate the infant to breathe.

Wrap the newborn in a blanket and cover its head. Repeat the suctioning as is necessary and continue to stimulate the newborn, by rubbing the back or flicking the soles if he or she is not yet breathing. If the newborn does not begin to breathe or continues to have breathing difficulty after 1 minute, the First Responder must consider the need for the following additional measures:

1. Ensure an open and patent airway.

2. Ventilate at a rate of 40 breaths per minute.

3. Reassess after 1 minute.

4. If the heart rate is less than 80 beats per minute, a second rescuer should perform chest compressions.

Postdelivery care of the mother should include keeping contact with the mother throughout the process. Remember to be attentive to her emotional as well as physical needs. Monitor the mother's respirations and pulse. Keep in mind that delivery is an exhausting procedure. Replace blood-soaked sheets and blankets, taking body substance isolation precautions and following your agency's exposure control plan. Finally, congratulate the family and your crew for helping bring a healthy child into the world!

REVIEW QUESTIONS

1. The vagina and lower part of the uterus are called the:
   A. placenta.
   B. birth canal.
   C. umbilicus.
   D. amniotic sac.

2. The organ through which the fetus exchanges nourishment and waste products during pregnancy is called the:
   A. placenta.
   B. birth canal.
   C. umbilical cord.
   D. amniotic sac.

3. The fetus's lifeline through which nourishment is received while in the uterus is called the:
   A. placenta.
   B. birth canal.
   C. umbilical cord.
   D. amniotic sac.

4. When the infant's presenting part bulges out of the vagina, this is called:
   A. placenta previa.
   B. crowning.
   C. the bag of waters.
   D. bearing down.

5. The muscular contractions of the uterus, beginning with the first uterine contraction and ending with the delivery of the placenta is called:
   A. a bloody show.
   B. crowning.
   C. labor.
   D. afterbirth.

6. The delivery of the products of conception very early in pregnancy is called:
   A. a multiple abortion.
   B. a miscarrage.
   C. labor.
   D. none of the above.

7. An indication of imminent delivery would be:
   A. labor pain.
   B. the urge to urinate.
   C. crowning.
   D. low back pain.

8. What questions should the First Responder ask to determine if delivery is imminent?
   A. What is your due date?
   B. Any chance of multiple births?
   C. Any bleeding or discharge?
   D. All of the above.

9. What is the relevance of asking if the patient feels as if she is having a bowel movement?
   A. Increasing pressure in the birth canal indicates that birth is imminent.
   B. The mother should be allowed to go to the bathroom prior to the birth.
   C. Extra pads will be required to clean up.
   D. This is an indication of multiple births.

10. If crowning is present, the First Responder should prepare for a prehospital delivery. The BSI required for a delivery includes:
    A. eye protection and mouth protection.
    B. disposable gloves.
    C. a gown to keep your uniform clean.
    D. all of the above.

11. A prehospital delivery is:
    A. a high potential for the spread of bloodborne pathogens.
    B. a very low potential for infection and disease spread.
    C. an extreme health hazard and to be avoided at all costs.
    D. all of the above.

12. If delivery is imminent and the First Responder is going to assist the mother in a prehospital delivery, after donning body substance isolation precautions the next step would be to:
    A. apply BSI to the mother.
    B. administer oxygen to the mother.
    C. have the mother lie on her back with her knees drawn up and legs spread apart.
    D. place the palm of your hand on top of the delivering baby's head and exert gentle pressure.

13. During a prehospital delivery, when the infant's head appears, the First Responder should:
    A. mark down the time of delivery.
    B. place the palm of the hand on top of the delivering baby's head and exert very gentle pressure.
    C. cut the umbilical cord.
    D. allow the mother to see the infant.

14. If the amniotic sac does not break or has not broken during a prehospital delivery, the First Responder should:
    A. tear it with his or her fingers and push it away from the infant's head.
    B. quickly cut the sac with a large sharp knife.
    C. ignore it as it will ultimately fall off.
    D. none of the above.

15. As the infant's head is being born, if the First Responder discovers that the umbilical cord is wrapped around the infant's neck, he or she should:
    A. call for an ALS unit.

B. attempt to slip the cord over the infant's head and shoulder.

C. allow the infant to put pressure on the cord while in the birth canal.

D. all of the above.

16. After the infant's head is born, the First Responder should support the head. Next suction:

A. the nose, then the mouth.

B. the mother's oropharynx.

C. the mouth, then the nostrils.

D. as little as possible.

17. Suctioning should be done with:

A. a rigid-tip Yankauer.

B. a bulb syringe.

C. a soft 18 french catheter.

D. the end of the suctioning tubing.

18. When the umbilical cord stops pulsating after the infant is delivered, the First Responder should:

A. remove it.

B. tie it with gauze between the mother and the infant.

C. start CPR compressions immediately.

D. transport the patient immediately.

19. If immediately after delivery the infant doesn't cry or breathe, the First Responder should:

A. call for transport immediately.

B. place the infant on the mother's abdomen.

C. try rubbing the baby's back or flicking the soles of its feet.

D. hold a newborn upside down by the legs to stimulate.

20. The mother will have vaginal bleeding following the delivery. Up to _____ of blood loss is well tolerated by the mother following delivery.

A. 100 to 300 mL

B. 300 to 500 mL

C. 500 to 700 mL

D. 700 to 900 mL

ANSWERS WITH RATIONALE

1. B. The vagina and lower part of the uterus is called the birth canal. Other terms are defined in the next three answers.

2. A. The organ through which the fetus exchanges nourishment and waste products during pregnancy is called the placenta. Other terms are defined in the next two answers.

3. C. The fetus's lifeline through which nourishment is received while in the uterus is called the placenta. The last term is defined in the next answer.

4. B. When the infant's presenting part bulges out of the vagina, this is called crowning. When the placenta itself exits first, this is called placenta previa. The bag of waters is the amniotic sac.

5. C. The muscular contractions of the uterus, beginning with the first uterine contraction and ending with the delivery of the placenta, is called labor. Crowning was defined in answer 4. Afterbirth is the placenta delivery, and a bloody show comes prior to delivery as an indication that birth is imminent and the infant has entered the birth canal.

6. B. The delivery of the products of conception very early in pregnancy is called a miscarrage. Labor is defined in answer 5.

7. C. An indication of imminent delivery is crowning. Labor pain starts early and may last for 12 hours prior to delivery being imminent in a first pregnancy. Some women experience low back pain from pressure on the nerves in the back during pregnancy.

8. D. What questions should the First Responder ask to determine if delivery is imminent? All of them are helpful: What is your due date? Any chance of multiple births? Any bleeding or discharge?

9. A. As the baby moves farther down the birth canal, pressure is exerted on the rectum causing the feeling of needing to have a bowel movement. This is an indication birth may by imminent. Do not allow the mother to go to the bathroom prior to the birth as the infant may end up delivered into the toilet! The feeling of having a bowel movement is not necessarily an indication of multiple births.

10. D. If crowning is present, the First Responder should prepare for a prehospital delivery. Don your body substance isolation equipment, which includes eye protection and mouth protection, disposable gloves, and a gown to keep your uniform clean.

11. A. A prehospital delivery is a high risk for the exposure to bloodborne pathogens, due to the potential for blood splattering. That is why gloves, goggles, and a gown should be worn.

12. C. If delivery is imminent and the First Responder is going to assist the mother in a prehospital delivery, after donning body substance isolation precautions the next step would be to have the mother lie on her back with her knees drawn up and legs spread apart. It is not necessary to administer oxygen to the mother unless you suspect a complication or hypoperfusion (shock).

13. B. During a prehospital delivery, when the infant's head appears the First Responder should place the palm of the hand on top of the delivering baby's head and exert very gentle pressure. Do not cut the umbilical cord at this early time, and it would not yet be possible to allow the mother to see the infant.

14. A. If the amniotic sac does not break or has not broken during a prehospital delivery, the First Responder should tear it with his or her fingers and push it away from the infant's head. Do not cut the sac quickly with a large, sharp knife, as you may injure the infant. If you ignore it, the infant will suffocate.

15. B. As the infant's head is being born, if the First Responder discovers that the umbilical cord is wrapped around the infant's neck, he or she should attempt to slip the cord over the infant's shoulder. You do not want the infant to put pressure on the cord while in the birth canal.

16. C. After the infant's head is born, the First Responder should support the head. Next suction the mouth and then the nostrils. Suctioning the nose first could cause the infant to gasp and aspirate the mucus in the mouth.

17. B. Suctioning should be done with a bulb syringe. A soft 18 french catheter would be too large, and the rigid tip is too dangerous for the infant's small mouth and nose.

18. B. When the umbilical cord stops pulsating after the infant is delivered, the First Responder should tie it with gauze between the mother and the infant. First Responders do not remove the cord surgically.

19. C. If immediately after delivery the infant does not cry or breathe, the First Responder should try rubbing the baby's back or flicking the soles of its feet. Never hold a newborn upside down by the legs for stimulation, as you may drop the child.

20. B. The mother will have vaginal bleeding following delivery. Up to 300 to 500 mL of blood loss is well tolerated by the mother following delivery.

6-2 Infants and Children

DOT OBJECTIVES

Cognitive Objectives

At the completion of this lesson, the First Responder student will be able to:

6-2.1 Describe differences in anatomy and physiology of the infant, child, and adult patient.

6-2.2 Describe assessment of the infant or child.

6-2.3 Indicate various causes of respiratory emergencies in infants and children.

6-2.4 Summarize emergency medical care strategies for respiratory distress and respiratory failure/arrest in infants and children.

6-2.5 List common causes of seizures in infants and children.

6-2.6 Describe management of seizures in the infant and child patient.

6-2.7 Discuss emergency medical care of the infant and child trauma patient.

6-2.8 Summarize the signs and symptoms of possible child abuse and neglect.

6-2.9 Describe the medical–legal responsibilities in suspected child abuse.

6-2.10 Recognize need for First Responder debriefing following a difficult infant or child transport.

Affective Objectives

At the completion of this lesson, the First Responder student will be able to:

6-2.11 Attend to the feelings of the family when dealing with an ill or injured infant or child.

6-2.12 Understand the provider's own emotional response to caring for infants or children.

6-2.13 Demonstrate a caring attitude towards infants and children with illness or injury who require emergency medical services.

6-2.14 Place the interests of the infant or child with an illness or injury as the foremost consideration when making any and all patient care decisions.

6-2.15 Communicate with empathy to infants and children with an illness or injury, as well as with family members and friends of the patient.

Psychomotor Objectives

At the completion of this lesson, the First Responder student will be able to:

6-2.16 Demonstrate assessment of the infant and child.

QUICK REVIEW The First Responder should become familiar with the anatomical and physiological differences between the infant, child, and adult patient. There are many differences between children and adults. Basically, children are not simply small adults and should not be evaluated or treated as such. Some of the differences between adult and child patients are described next.

A child's or infant's small airways are often blocked by secretions and airway swelling. The tongue is large relative to the small airways and can block the airway in an unresponsive infant or child. When opening the airway in an infant it is important not to hyperextend the neck, as this may kink and close the airway. Because infants are primarily nose breathers, the importance of suctioning a secretion-filled nasopharynx cannot be overstated.

Children can compensate well for short periods of time when confronted with respiratory problems and hypoperfusion (shock). They compensate by increasing breathing rate and increasing the effort of breathing. Although they compensate well, they crash easily or rapidly decompensate from respiratory muscle fatigue. Finally, infants and children have an increased risk of hypothermia. Due to the large surface area of the head, be sure an infant's or child's head is covered when outside.

When conducting an assessment, be sure to involve the parents in your assessment and management of their infant or child. Remember that agitated parents mean an agitated child, and calm parents mean a calm child. The general impression of a child's wellness can be obtained by paying attention to overall appearance. Observe for mental status, effort of breathing, color, quality of cry or speech, emotional state (i.e., is he or she crying or showing other signs of fright or upset?), and muscle tone or body position.

Evaluate interaction with the environment and the child's parents. Ask yourself the following questions:

1. Is the behavior normal for a child of this age?

2. Is the child playing or moving about?

3. Is the child attentive as you enter the room, and is he or she able to recognize his or her parents?

Your assessment should begin from across the room by observing for the mechanism of injury and assessing the patient's surroundings. Rapid assessment of respiratory problems is especially important in a child. For that reason the First Responder's ability to do a respiratory assessment should include:

- Chest expansion and symmetry

- Effort of breathing

- Nasal flaring

- Stridor or crowing

- Retractions

- Grunting

- Respiratory rate

- Comparison between brachial and femoral pulses

- Comparison between central (core of the body) and distal (extremity) pulses

- Assessment of skin color, temperature, and condition

Common respiratory problems in infants and children include partial airway obstruction, respiratory distress, respiratory failure, and circulatory failure.

- In partial airway obstruction in an alert and sitting patient, there is good peripheral perfusion, a pink color, and retractions and stridor on inspiration.

- In complete airway obstruction in a patient with an altered mental status or a partial obstruction with cyanosis, the children are unable to cry or speak.

- Respiratory distress, which often precedes respiratory failure, is indicated when the patient has a respiratory rate greater than 60 in infants or greater than 30 to 40 in children. Shows nasal flaring, intercostal supraclavicular and subcostal retractions, stridor, cyanosis, grunting, and altered mental status.

- Respiratory failure leading to respiratory arrest is indicated when the breathing rate is less than 10 per minute in a child and less than 20 per minute in an infant. The patient exhibits limp muscle tone, or is unresponsive, with a slower or absent heart rate and weak or absent pulse as well as cyanosis.

- Circulatory failure that is uncorrected is a common cause of cardiac arrest in infants and children. The signs and symptoms of circulatory failure include an increased heart rate, unequal central and distal pulses, poor skin perfusion, and mental status changes.

The role of the First Responder in a respiratory emergency would be to complete the First Responder assessment, which includes a size-up prior to initiating care, an initial assessment on all patients, a physical exam as needed, and an ongoing assessment. The First Responder also needs to be able to provide mouth-to-mask or barrier device ventilations and to observe the heart rate.

In a circulatory failure the First Responder's role is to complete the First Responder assessment. This involves providing a complete scene size-up prior to initiating emergency medical care. Be sure to complete an initial assessment on all patients and support oxygenation and ventilation while observing for cardiac arrest.

Seizures should be considered potentially life threatening. The causes of seizures include the following:

- Fever

- Infections

- Poisoning

- Low blood sugar

- Trauma

- Decreased levels of oxygen

- Unknown causes in children

The role of the First Responder in the management of seizures involves completing an assessment that includes a scene size-up prior to starting emergency medical care, an initial assessment on all patients, a physical exam as needed, an ongoing assessment, and observing and describing the seizure. The First Responder's role also involves comforting, calming, and reassuring the patient while awaiting additional EMS resources. Be sure to protect the patient from the environment. Ask bystanders (except parents) to leave the area, observe patency of the airway, and place the patient in the recovery position if there is no possibility of spinal trauma. In a seizure the First Responder should not restrain the patient.

Do not put anything in the patient's mouth, as he or she may undergo further injury or possibly aspirate the foreign body. Always have suction available for seizure patients, due to the volume of secretions. Finally, if the patient is bluish, make sure that the airway is open and provide artificial ventilation if required.

Injuries are the leading cause of death in infants and children. Blunt injury is more common than penetrating injury. The typical injury patterns found in infants and children include:

- Motor vehicle crashes (i.e., unrestrained motor vehicle passengers have head and neck injuries, restrained passengers have abdominal and lower spine injuries). Infant booster seats are often improperly fastened, resulting in head and neck injuries. Children are also injured when struck while riding a bicycle, resulting in head, spine, and abdominal injuries. Children are also injured by vehicles when struck as pedestrians, resulting in, for example, abdominal injury with internal bleeding, a painful, swollen, deformed extremity, and head injury.

- Falls from height—frequently from diving into shallow water, resulting in head and neck injuries.

- Burns, sports injuries to the head and neck, and child abuse and neglect.

Some injuries can be averted or better managed when the First Responder has a knowledge of the effects of trauma to specific body systems. The head is proportionally larger and more easily injured. The single most important maneuver is to ensure an open airway by means of the jaw thrust. The chest is very pliable, due to soft ribs. There may be significant injuries without external signs. Toddlers have been known to have tire tracks across their chest: although there were no rib fractures, severe internal contusions were present. The abdomen is a more common site of injury in children than in adults. It is often a source of hidden injury.

The role of the First Responder when confronted with an infant or child who has experienced trauma is to complete a scene size-up before initiating emergency medical care. Complete an initial assessment on all patients and a physical exam as needed. The ongoing assessment should be done on all patients as is appropriate based on their condition. The First Responder should be sure to assure airway position and patency by using a jaw thrust, suction as necessary with a large-bore suction catheter, provide spinal stabilization, stabilize extremity injuries manually, and comfort, calm, and reassure the patient while awaiting additional EMS resources.

Child abuse is defined as improper or excessive action so as to injure or cause harm to a child. Neglect is the giving of insufficient attention or respect to someone who has a claim to that attention. As a First Responder you must be aware of a situation to be able to recognize the problem of child abuse or neglect. The signs and symptoms of abuse include:

- Multiple bruises in various stages of healing

- Injury inconsistent with the mechanism described

- Suspect patterns of injury (i.e., cigarette burns, whip marks, and hand prints)

- Repeated calls to the same address

- Fresh burns inconsistent with the history presented or untreated (i.e., scalding, glove, or dip pattern)

- Parents seem inappropriately unconcerned

- Conflicting stories

- Fear on the part of the child to discuss how the injury occurred

- Central nervous system injuries (i.e., shaken baby syndrome), exhibiting severe internal injuries, unresponsiveness, and/or seizure activity, and no evidence of external injuries

- Signs and symptoms of neglect (i.e., lack of adult supervision, malnourished-appearing children, unsafe living environment, untreated chronic illness, untreated soft tissue injuries)

Do not accuse anyone of child abuse or neglect in the field. This may only delay getting appropriate medical care for the patient. Your role is to report the objective information to the transporting unit. The First Responder should be aware of the reporting requirements required by state law and local regulations. Be careful to report exactly what you see and hear, not what you think.

The First Responder should learn when it is most appropriate to call for a debriefing following a difficult infant or child transport. Take inventory of the resources within your community and/or state for critical incident debriefing of prehospital personnel.

REVIEW QUESTIONS

1. Why should the First Responder become familiar with the anatomical and physiological differences between the infant, child, and adult patient?
   A. Because children are small adults and should be treated as such.
   B. There are many important differences between children and adults.
   C. Knowledge of pathophysiology is needed to diagnose the problem.
   D. All of the above.

2. Each of the following are differences between the adult and child patient except:
   A. a child or infant's small airways are often blocked by secretions and airway swelling.
   B. the tongue is large relative to the small airways and can block the airway in an unresponsive infant or child.

C. when opening the airway in an infant it is important to hyperextend the neck.

D. infants are primarily nose breathers, so suctioning a secretion-filled nasopharynx is important.

3. Children can compensate well for short periods of time when confronted with respiratory problems and hypoperfusion (shock). They compensate by:

A. increasing breathing rate and increasing the effort of breathing.

B. decreasing breathing rate and decreasing the effort of breathing.

C. decreasing their pulse rate and increasing their blood pressure.

D. none of the above.

4. Since infants and children have an increased risk of hypothermia, the First Responder should:

A. consider any altered level of consciousness from cold exposure.

B. be sure to cover the patient's head when out in the cold weather.

C. determine if the patient has eaten within the past hour.

D. all of the above.

5. Why should the First Responder involve parents in the assessment and management of infants and children?

A. The law requires you to involve the parent in treatment.

B. They always know what is wrong with the child.

C. Calm parents mean a calm child.

D. all of the above.

6. The general impression of the child's wellness can be obtained by paying attention to their overall appearance. The First Responder should observe for:

A. mental status.

B. effort of breathing.

C. quality of cry or speech.

D. all of the above.

7. The First Responder's respiratory assessment should include all of the following except:

A. chest expansion and symmetry.

B. effort of breathing.

C. capillary refill.

D. observing nasal flaring.

8. One way to assess the circulatory status of a child is to:
   A. observe for retractions.
   B. listen for stridor or crowing.
   C. compare brachial pulse to the femoral pulse.
   D. none of the above.

9. Common respiratory problems in infants and children include:
   A. partial airway obstruction.
   B. respiratory distress.
   C. respiratory failure.
   D. all of the above.

10. Respiratory distress is indicated when the patient has a respiratory rate greater than:
    A. 60 in infants.
    B. 40 to 50 in children.
    C. 80 in infants.
    D. none of the above.

11. Respiratory failure is indicated when the breathing rate is less than:
    A. 20 per minute in a child.
    B. 10 per minute in a child.
    C. 30 per minute in an infant.
    D. all of the above.

12. If your child patient exhibits limp muscle tone, or is unresponsive, with a slower or absent heart rate and weak or absent pulse as well as cyanosis, the problem probably is:
    A. partial obstruction.
    B. respiratory distress.
    C. respiratory failure.
    D circulatory failure.

13. The causes of seizures include the following:
    A. fever and infections.
    B. poisoning and low blood sugar.
    C. trauma and decreased levels of oxygen.
    D. all of the above.

14. The role of the First Responder in the management of seizures involves completing all of the following except:
   A. an assessment that includes a scene size-up prior to starting emergency medical care.
   B. an initial assessment on only the most serious patients.
   C. a physical exam as needed.
   D. an ongoing assessment and observing and describing the seizure.

15. The First Responder's role with a seizure patient also involves comforting, calming, and reassuring the patient while awaiting additional EMS resources. In addition, the First Responder should:
   A. be sure to protect the patient from the environment.
   B. ask parents to leave the area.
   C. be sure to reduce the patency of the airway.
   D. all of the above.

16. Why shouldn't the First Responder place something in the seizure patient's mouth?
   A. It can cause spinal trauma.
   B. The patient may further injure himself or herself.
   C. It may not be sterile.
   D. all of the above.

17. Injuries are the leading cause of death in infants and children. What type of injuries are most common?
   A. Blunt injury
   B. Elevator injuries
   C. Penetrating injury
   D. None of the above

18. Typical causes of injury found in infants and children include:
   A. motor vehicle crashes.
   B. falls from heights.
   C. burns.
   D. all of the above.

19. When a child is struck by an automobile while riding a bike, he or she often will injure the:
   A. face and shoulders.
   B. neck and abdominal area.
   C. head and buttock.
   D. none of the above.

20. The single most important maneuver to treat a child with unconsciousness from trauma is the:
    A. jaw thrust.
    B. mouth-to-mask ventilation.
    C. doll's-eye maneuver.
    D. Heimlich maneuver.

21. A frequent cause of an injury from a fall in children is due to:
    A. suicide.
    B. a fractured hip.
    C. a deep dive in a shallow pool.
    D. none of the above.

22. Because the child's chest is still very pliable:
    A. there may be significant injuries without external signs.
    B. the ribs break very easily.
    C. the internal organs are well protected from injury.
    D. all of the above.

23. As a First Responder you must be aware of a situation to be able to recognize the problem of child abuse or neglect. The signs and symptoms of abuse include all of the following except:
    A. multiple bruises in various stages of healing.
    B. injury inconsistent with the mechanism described.
    C. suspect patterns of injury, such as the knees and elbows.
    D. repeated calls to the same address.

24. Shaken baby syndrome may exhibit as:
    A. severe internal injuries.
    B. unresponsiveness and/or seizure activity.
    C. no evidence of external injuries.
    D. all of the above.

25. Why should the First responder avoid accusing anyone of child abuse or neglect in the field?
    A. This may only delay patients getting to see appropriate medical care.
    B. Your role is to report the subjective information to the transporting unit.
    C. It is against the law in some jurisdictions.
    D. All of the above.

1. B. The First Responder should become familiar with the anatomical and physiological differences between infant, child, and adult patients. There are many differences between children and adults, so young patients should not be treated like little adults. Knowledge of pathophysiology is not necessary, as the First Responder does not "diagnose" the problem.

2. C. Each of the following are differences between the adult and child patient: a child or infant's small airways are often blocked by secretions and airway swelling, the tongue is large relative to the small airways and can block the airway in an unresponsive infant or child, and infants are primarily nose breathers. It is inappropriate to hyperextend the child's neck, as you may actually kink it closed.

3. A. Children can compensate well for short periods of time when confronted with respiratory problems and hypoperfusion (shock). They compensate by increasing their breathing rate and increasing the effort of breathing.

4. B. Since infants and children have an increased risk of hypothermia, the First Responder should be sure to cover the patient's head when out in cold weather. Determining if the patient has eaten within the past hour is part of the SAMPLE history but not relevant to hyperthermia. We do not automatically assume that an altered level of consciousness is hypothermia.

5. C. Why should the First Responder involve parents in the assessment and management of infants and children? Because calm parents mean a calm child. No, it is not the law that the parents must assess and manage their own children. Do not confuse who provides the treatment with consent for treatment of a minor.

6. D. The general impression of the child's wellness can be obtained by paying attention to their overall appearance. The First Responder should observe for mental status, effort of breathing, and quality of cry or speech.

7. C. The First Responder's respiratory assessment should include chest expansion and symmetry, effort of breathing, and observing nasal flaring. Capillary refill is a quick means of assessing the circulatory status of the patient.

8. C. One way to assess the circulatory status of a child is to compare brachial pulse to femoral pulse. This will give you an assessment of the central versus peripheral circulation. Listening for stridor or crowing and observing for retractions are part of the respiratory assessment.

9. D. Common respiratory problems in infants and children include partial airway obstruction, respiratory distress, and respiratory failure.

10. A. Respiratory distress is indicated when an infant has a respiratory rate greater than 60.

11. B. Respiratory failure is indicated when the breathing rate is less than 10 per minute in a child.

12. C. If your child patient exhibits limp muscle tone or is unresponsive, with a slower or absent heart rate and weak or absent pulse as well as cyanosis, the problem probably is respiratory failure.

13. D. The causes of seizures include the following: fever and infections, poisoning and low blood sugar, and trauma and decreased levels of oxygen.

14. B. The role of the First Responder in the management of seizures involves completing all of the following: an assessment that includes a scene size-up prior to starting emergency medical care, an initial assessment, a physical exam as needed, an ongoing assessment, and observing and describing the seizure. The initial assessment should be completed on all patients, not just serious cases.

15. A. The First Responder's role with a seizure patient also involves comforting, calming, and reassuring the patient while awaiting additional EMS resources. In addition, the First Responder should be sure to protect the patient from the environment. We do not ask parents to leave the area.

16. B. Why shouldn't the First Responder place something in the seizure patient's mouth? The patient may further injure himself or herself. It can also become an obstruction and cause the patient to vomit and possibly to aspirate.

17. A. Injuries are the leading cause of death in infants and children. Blunt injuries are the most common.

18. D. Typical injuries found in infants and children include motor vehicle crashes, falls from heights, and burns.

19. B. When a child is struck by an automobile while riding on a bike, he or she will often injure the head, neck, and abdomen.

20. A. The single most important maneuver in treating a child with unconsciousness from trauma is the jaw thrust maneuver to

open the airway. Doll's-eyes maneuver is never done in the field, and the Heimlich maneuver is used on an obstructed airway.

21. C. The most frequent cause of an injury from a fall in children is due to a deep dive in a shallow pool. Suicides are increasing in adolescents but not the most common cause of falls. A fractured hip injury from a fall is common in the elderly.

22. A. Because a child's chest is still very pliable, there may be significant injuries without external signs. The ribs do not break very easily.

23. C. As a First Responder you must be aware of a situation to be able to recognize the problem of child abuse or neglect. The signs and symptoms of abuse include all of the following: multiple bruises in various stages of healing, injury inconsistent with the mechanism described, repeated calls to the same address, and suspect patterns such as cigarette burns and whip marks. Most children commonly have bruises on the knees and elbows from falls in the playground.

24. D. Shaken baby syndrome may exhibit as severe internal injuries, unresponsiveness and/or seizure activity, and no evidence of external injuries.

25. A. Accusing someone of child abuse or neglect in the field may only delay the patient getting to see appropriate medical care. Your role is to report the objective, not subjective, information to the transporting unit.

LESSON

7-1 EMS Operations

DOT
OBJECTIVES

Cognitive Objectives

At the completion of this lesson, the First Responder student will be able to:

7-1.1 Discuss the medical and non-medical equipment needed to respond to a call.

7-1.2 List the phases of an out-of-hospital call.

7-1.3 Discuss the role of the First Responder in extrication.

7-1.4 List various methods of gaining access to the patient.

7-1.5 Distinguish between simple and complex access.

7-1.6 Describe what the First Responder should do if there is reason to believe that there is a hazard at the scene.

7-1.7 State the role the First Responder should do if there is reason to believe that there is a hazard at the scene.

7-1.8 Describe the criteria for a multiple casualty situation.

7-1.9 Discuss the role of the First Responder in the multiple casualty situation.

7-1.10 Summarize the components of basic triage.

7-1.11 Explain the rationale for having the unit prepared to respond.

7-1.12 Given a scenario of a mass casualty incident, perform triage.

One important role of the First Responder is to assure that the appropriate equipment is carried on the unit and to the patient's side as well as checking the medical and nonmedical equipment each shift. Checking equipment is part of the six phases of a call:

1. Preparation for the call

2. Dispatch

3. Enroute to the scene

4. Arrival at the scene

5. Transferring the patient to the ambulance

6. Postrun

Equipment will need to be checked and maintained, restocked after each call and repaired as deficiencies are encountered. The medical equipment includes: basic supplies, airways, suction equipment, artificial ventilation devices and basic wound care supplies. The nonmedical equipment includes personal safety equipment to satisfy local, state, or federal OSHA standards (e.g., gloves, goggles, turnout coats, helmets; personal protective equipment). Other aspects of preparation include having sufficient numbers of trained personnel.

The next phase of a call is dispatch, which involves central access, preferably a 911 or enhanced 911 system with 24-hour availability. The best dispatch centers have Emergency Medical Dispatchers (EMDs) who are properly trained to provide prearrival instructions and obtain the nature of the call, name of the patient, location and callback number of the caller, location of the patient, number of patients, and severity and other special problems.

En route to the scene the first responder must always wear his or her seat belt and drive with due regard for the safety of all others on the road. Be sure to notify dispatch that you are enroute and take note of the essential call information, including the nature and location of the call.

Upon arrival at the scene, notify dispatch that you have arrived at the patient's side and begin your size-up of the scene. The size-up includes utilizing the appropriate body substance isolation (BSI) prior to patient contact. Evaluate the scene for hazards to yourself, your crew members and the patient. Make sure that the emergency vehicle is parked in a safe location off the road. Be sure it is safe to approach the patient and determine if an emergent move will be required to move the patient quickly to a safe spot.

In addition to sizing up the total number of patients and the need for additional help or assistance at the scene, the mechanism of injury or nature of illness should be evaluated. If the situation is a medical or traumatic complaint, the first responder will need to determine the number of patients and if the incident is a multiple casualty incident (MCI). This may require additional help and the need for triage. In situations where trauma has occurred, cervical collars and long spineboards may be needed once you suspect a potential back injruy.

The next phase of a call involves transferring the patient to the ambulance. The First Responder should offer to assist the ambulance crew in preparing the patient for transport. Also assist the ambulance crew with lifting and moving using the guidelines discussed in Chapter 5.

The last phase of the call involves the postrun activities, such as the completion of the prehospital care report (PCR), preparing the unit for the next call by cleaning and disinfecting equipment, refueling as needed, and restocking any disposable supplies used on the call.

Many communities have access to air medical evacuation. Therefore, it is important that you know your local capabilities for air transport, when and whom to call, and what types of mission they will accept. Operational reasons for using a helicopter include:

1. Ground transportation to the appropriate critical care facility will exceed 30 minutes.

2. The helicopter can be airborne with a proper crew and can be at the scene quicker than an ambulance can transport the patient(s) to the nearest hospital.

3. Extrication time at the scene is estimated to exceed 20 minutes.

4. Ground transportation could be hazardous to the patient (possible reasons are weather conditions and confirmed spinal cord injury).

5. A helicopter landing site is available.

6. A multiple-casualty incident threatens to overload local capabilities.

7. The situation is one of difficult access, such as wilderness rescue, or access or egress is impeded at the scene by road conditions, weather, traffic, or search and rescue situations.

8. A patient needs a higher level of ALS care than your agency can provide.

There is a high priority for rapid transport if the patient was injured in a collision in which evidence of any one of the following high-energy conditions exists or patient exam reveals that any of the following abnormal vital signs or physical findings exist:

- Fall of 15 feet or more

- Patient struck by a vehicle moving at 20 mph or faster

- Patient ejected from a vehicle

- Vehicle rollover with unrestrained passengers

- High-speed crash with 20 inches or more front-end deformity

- Deformity into the passenger compartment of 15 inches or more

- Patient a survivor of a motor vehicle collision where a death occurred in the same vehicle

- Glasgow coma score (GCS) of 13 or less (the GCS may be used and taught in your regional EMS system; check with your service medical director)

- Trauma score (TS) of 14 or less (the TS may be used and taught in your regional EMS system. Check with your service medical director)

- Sustained pulse rate of 120 per minute or more

- Head trauma with altered level of consciousness or hemiplegia (inability to move one side of the body)

- Penetrating injuries of the head, neck, chest, abdomen, or groin

- Chest trauma with respiratory distress

- Two or more proximal long-bone fractures

- Amputations requiring reimplantation

- Facial/airway burns; burns of 15% body surface or greater

- Interhospital transfer of a critical patient

- Transport to a hyperbaric chamber

If air rescue is utilized in your community, you should be aware of how to locate a landing zone (LZ). Depending on the ship used, an area of 100 by 100 feet should be located which is clear of wires, towers, vehicles, people, and loose objects. The ground must be level and firm.

Finally, learn how to prepare patients for aeromedical evacuation and safety around the ship. Standing near a running helicopter can be extremely dangerous. Never go near the tail rotor since it spins so fast that you cannot see it spinning. Approach the helicopter only if instructed by the flight crew and approach from the front of the ship.

Fundamentals of Extrication

The First Responder's role is to administer necessary care to the patient before extrication and assure that the patient is removed so as to minimize further injury. Patient care should precede extrication unless delayed movement would endanger the life of the patient or First Responder. In some instances, the First Responders are also the rescue providers. A chain of command should be established to ensure patient care priorities.

Equipment is needed for the First Responder to provide personal and patient safety. Since First Responder safety is the number one priority, protective clothing should be worn. The next priority is patient safety, through informing him or her of the unique aspects of the extrication. Protect the patient from broken glass, sharp metal, and other hazards, including the environment.

Gaining access to the patient may be simple or complex. Simple access does not require the use of specialized equipment. Always try to open all doors to the vehicle prior to having rescue personnel utilize heavy tools to provide access through the doors. If the patient can unlock the doors and roll down windows, this will help you gain access.

Complex access will require the use of specialized tools and training. There are a number of training programs that can be taken to prepare for specialty rescue, such as:

1. Vehicle rescue

2. Water rescue

3. High-angle rescue, low-angle rescue , or rope rescue

4. Trench rescue

5. Confined-space rescue

Removal of the patient should be done by working closely with EMS providers. Be sure to maintain spine stabilization, complete the initial assessment, and then provide critical interventions.

The First Responder should be knowledgeable in the dangers of hazardous materials since this is becoming a more common problem. The primary concern is the First Responder crew as well as the patient and the public.

When approaching the scene the First Responder should attempt to identify the product from a safe location. Consider clues such as:

- Type of occupancy

- Container size and shape

- Placards that are present

- Shipping papers as well as using all your senses

General procedures the First Responder should consider include:

1. Parking upwind/hill from the incident, at a safe distance.

2. Keeping unnecessary people away from the area.

3. Isolating the area to keep people out. Only properly trained and outfitted rescue personnel should enter the scene.

4. Avoiding contact with the material.

5. Removing to a safe zone patients who are no risk to the First Responder.

6. Not entering a haz-mat area unless you are trained as a haz-mat technician.

Be careful to utilize multiple resources to identify the substance. Become familiar with the U.S. DOT Emergency Response Handbook as well as the OSHA and NFPA rules and publications on haz-mat.

The First Responder should be knowledgeable in aspects of basic triage at a multiple-casualty incident. *Triage* is a French word which means "to sort." There are three levels of triage categories: high, second, and low priority. Examples in each category are as follows:

- High priority: airway and breathing difficulties, uncontrolled or severe bleeding, and decreased mental status

- Second priority: burns without airway problems, major or multiple painful, swollen, deformed extremities, and back injuries

- Lowest priority: minor painful, swollen, deformed extremities, minor soft tissue injuries, and dead patients

The procedures with which the First Responder should be knowledgeable upon arrival at an MCI include:

1. Assign the most knowledgeable EMS provider on the scene to be the first triage officer until relieved by someone with higher training.

2. Confirm the incident and establish EMS command.

3. Request needed additional help.

4. Make sure that an initial assessment is performed for each patient.

5. Prepare a triage tag for each patient.

6. Assign available personnel and equipment to the priority one (highest-priority) patients.

7. Arrange that a triage officer remain at the scene to assign and coordinate personnel, supplies, and vehicles.

If you are told to respond to an already "declared" MCI, report to the command post and identify the Incident Commander so you can identify yourself and your level of training. Follow directions given to you from the Incident Commander.

1. Examples of nonmedical equipment needed to respond to a call include:
   A. helmets.
   B. gloves and goggles.
   C. turnout coats.
   D. all of the above.

2. All of the following are considered medical equipment except:
   A. bandages.
   B. turnout coat.
   C. suction unit.
   D. all of the above.

3. In an extrication the First Responder should:
   A. direct the operation of the rescue tools.
   B. assure that the patient is removed in a way to minimize injury.
   C. utilize the "jaws of life" for door removal.
   D. all of the above.

4. The six phases of a call include all of the following except:
   A. size-up.
   B. dispatch.
   C. preparation for a call.
   D. post run.

5. During the dispatch phase of a call the EMD must obtain:
   A. the nature of the call.
   B. the number of patients.
   C. a callback number for the caller.
   D. all of the above.

6. What type of access involves asking the patient to unlock the doors?
   A. Initial
   B. Simple
   C. Complex
   D. None of the above

7. Access requiring specialized hydraulic tools is called:
   A. initial.
   B. simple.

C. complex.

D. none of the above.

8. Your size-up of the scene should evaluate:

   A. where to park your vehicle.

   B. potential hazards to yourself.

   C. potential hazards to the patient.

   D. all of the above.

9. Clues to consider when attempting to identify a hazardous material include:

   A. placards on the vehicle.

   B. container size and shape.

   C. shipping papers.

   D. all of the above.

10. Which of the following is not a clue to consider in identifying a hazardous material?

    A. Type of occupancy

    B. The way the material tastes

    C. Shipping papers

    D. Placard on a vehicle

11. Operational reasons for using a helicopter include all of the following except:

    A. extrication time at the scene is estimated to exceed 20 minutes.

    B. the helicopter can be airborne with crew and be at the scene faster than an ambulance can transport to a hospital.

    C. the patient is in cardiac arrest.

    D. weather conditions and a confirmed spinal cord injury.

12. Physical findings that would cause a helicopter to respond include all of the following except:

    A. falls of 15 feet or more.

    B. a Glascow coma score over 13.

    C. a sustained pulse rate of 120 per minute.

    D. vehicle rollover with an unrestrained patient.

13. Before approaching a helicopter:

    A. wait for the crew to approve your approaching the ship.

    B. insist that the helicopter be turned off.

    C. motion the pilot with a bright white beam of light.

    D. all of the above.

14. The most dangerous approach to a running helicopter would be from the:
    A. rear area.
    B. front area.
    C. right side.
    D. left side.

15. Upon arrival at a hazardous materials incident the First Responder should:
    A. park downwind of the spill.
    B. avoid contact with the material.
    C. handle the product with care.
    D. all of the above.

ANSWERS WITH RATIONALE

1. D. Examples of nonmedical equipment needed to respond to a call include helmets, gloves, goggles, and turnout coats.

2. B. Bandages and a suction unit are considered medical equipment. A turnout coat is considered personal protective or rescue equipment.

3. B. In an extrication the First Responder should assure that the patient is removed in a way to minimize injury. This is the medical role of the inside rescuer, as are continuing a concerned dialogue and assessing the patient. The specifics of directing operation of the rescue tools and utilizing the "jaws of life" for door removal should be left up to the rescue personnel.

4. A. The six phases of a call are preparation for the call, dispatch, en route to the scene, arrival at the scene, transferring the patient to the ambulance, and postrun. Size-up is considered a part of the patient assessment process.

5. D. During the dispatch phase of a call the emergency medical dispatcher (EMD) must obtain the nature of the call, the number of patients, and a callback number for the caller.

6. B. Simple access involves asking the patient to unlock the doors. Complex access may involve dismantling a door or cutting through the floorboard of an overturned vehicle. *Initial access* is not a term commonly used.

7. C. Access requiring specialized hydraulic tools is called complex access. Simple access is defined in question 6.

8. D. Your size-up of the scene should evaluate where to park your vehicle, potential hazards to yourself, and potential hazards to the patient.

9. D. Clues to consider when attempting to identify a hazardous material include placards on the vehicle, the type of occupancy, shipping papers, and container size and shape.

10. B. The way the material tastes is dangerous and not a clue to consider in identifying a hazardous material. Clues to consider are listed in question 9.

11. C. Operational reasons for using a helicopter include: extrication time at the scene is estimated to exceed 20 minutes, the helicopter can be airborne with crew and be at the scene faster than an ambulance can transport to a hospital, and weather conditions and a confirmed spinal cord injury. Most helicopter programs do not plan to transport cardiac arrest victims unless they are hypothermic (low body temperature) arrests.

12. B. Physical findings that would cause your helicopter to respond include: falls of 15 feet or more, sustained pulse rate of 120 per minute, and vehicle rollover with an unrestrained patient. A patient with a Glascow coma score over 13 is not considered severe enough for a helicopter unless the person has associated trauma such as severe shock.

13. A. Before approaching a helicopter, wait for the crew to approve your approaching the ship. It is often impractable to insist that the helicopter be turned off. Never motion the pilot with a bright white beam of light, as it can severely affect his or her eyesight and ability to land the ship.

14. A. The most dangerous approach to a running helicopter is from the rear area. This is because the tail rotor spins so fast that it is often impossible to see and you could easily walk right into the rotor and be fatally injured.

15. B. Upon arrival at a hazardous materials incident, the First Responder should avoid contact with the material. Do not park downwind of the product, as you may easily become overcome with vapors from the product. Do not handle the product at all until it is identified and the proper precautions have been taken.

Automated External Defibrillation

**D O T
OBJECTIVES**

Cognitive Objectives:

At the completion of this lesson, the First Responder student will be able to:

1. List the indications for automated external defibrillation (AED).

2. List the contraindications for automated external defibrillation.

3. Explain the impact of age and weight on defibrillation.

4. Discuss the fundamentals of early defibrillation.

5. Explain the rationale for early defibrillation.

6. Explain that not all chest pain patients result in cardiac arrest and do not need to be attached to an automated external defibrillator.

7. Explain the importance of prehospital ACLS intervention if it is available.

8. Explain the importance of urgent transport to a facility with Advanced Cardiac Life Support if it is not available in the prehospital setting.

9. Discuss the various types of automated external defibrillators.

10. Differentiate between the fully automated and the semiautomated defibrillator.

11. Discuss the procedures that must be taken into consideration for standard operations of the various types of automated external defibrillators.

12. State the reasons for assuring that the patient is pulseless and apneic when using the automated external defibrillator.

13. Discuss the circumstances which may result in inappropriate shocks.

14. Explain the considerations for interruption of CPR, when using the automated external defibrillator.

15. Discuss the advantages and disadvantages of automated external defibrillators.

16. Summarize the speed of operation of automated external defibrillation.

17. Discuss the use of remote defibrillation through adhesive pads.

18. Discuss the special considerations for rhythm monitoring.

19. List the steps in the operation of the automated external defibrillator.

20. Discuss the standard of care that should be used to provide care to a patient with persistent ventricular fibrillation and no available ACLS.

21. Differentiate between the single rescuer and multi-rescuer care with an automated external defibrillator.

22. Explain the reason for pulses not being checked between shocks with an automated external defibrillator.

23. Discuss the importance of coordinating ACLS trained providers with personnel using automated external defibrillators.

24. Discuss the importance of post-resuscitation care.

25. List the components of post-resuscitation care.

26. Explain the importance of frequent practice with the automated external defibrillator.

27. Discuss the need to complete the Automated Defibrillator: Operator's Shift Checklist.

28. Discuss the role of the American Heart Association (AHA) in the use of automated external defibrillation.

29. Explain the role medical direction plays in the use of automated external defibrillation.

30. State the reasons why a case review should be completed following the use of the automated external defibrillator.

31. Discuss the components that should be included in a case review.

32. Discuss the goal of quality improvement in automated external defibrillation.

33. Define the function of all controls on an automated external defibrillator, and describe event documentation and battery defibrillator maintenance.

Affective Objectives:

At the completion of this lesson, the First Responder student will be able to:

34. Defend the reasons for obtaining initial training in automated external defibrillation and the importance of continuing education.

35. Defend the reason for maintenance of automated external defibrillators.

Psychomotor Objectives:

At the completion of this lesson, the First Responder student will be able to:

36. Demonstrate the application and operation of the automated external defibrillator.

37. Demonstrate the maintenance of an automated external defibrillator.

38. Demonstrate the assessment and documentation of patient response to the automated external defibrillator.

39. Demonstrate the skills necessary to complete the Automated Defibrillator: Operator's Shift Checklist.

As you are already aware, defibrillation is an important link in the American Heart Association's chain of survival. The survival of a patient in cardiac arrest depends on each link being in place. If you are trained and authorized to use an automated external defibrillator, you possess a truly lifesaving skill.

Automated external defibrillation is relatively easy to perform. You will be given initial training and continuing education with skill proficiency exams. Your EMS system will have a medical director to oversee the system. A quality improvement program will also be formed to monitor the use of AEDs.

One of the great benefits of the automated external defibrillator is the ease of use and the relatively short time it takes to administer lifesaving shocks to a patient in cardiac arrest. Although there are benefits, other areas require caution. The AED must be operated in accordance with medical control guidelines. The units must be maintained properly and checked on every shift using the AED checklist. Something as simple as a dead battery eliminates the lifesaving potential of the AED.

There are two types of automated external defibrillators: automated defibrillators operated without action by the First Responder, and semiautomated defibrillators, which prompt the First Responder with verbal instructions. Some defibrillators provide the ability to observe the heart rhythm on a viewing screen.

AEDs are able to interpret the patient's cardiac rhythm by the use of a computer microprocessor within the unit. There are two rhythms that will require a shock:

- *Ventricular fibrillation* (V-Fib). This is a chaotic, disorganized heart rhythm. The heart normally contracts forcefully in a specific order. With V-Fib, the electrical impulses throughout the heart fire randomly, producing a quivering rather than a pumping action. V-Fib will not produce a pulse.

- *Ventricular tachycardia* (V-Tach). This rhythm is more organized than V-Fib but much less efficient than the normal heart rhythm. This rhythm may or may not produce a pulse.

It is not actually necessary to identify each rhythm, the AED will do that for you. There are several steps that you must take to assure proper operation of the AED and the safety of your patient. In general:

- The AED must be properly maintained and have charged batteries at all times.

- The AED must be attached only to patients who are unresponsive, pulseless, and nonbreathing.

- No one may touch the patient while the AED is analyzing the heart rhythm and when shocks are being delivered.

- Defibrillation is more effective than CPR. Stopping CPR to defibrillate is not only acceptable but beneficial to the patient.

If defibrillation is required, CPR will also be required. CPR must be discontinued when the AED is analyzing the rhythm and while the shock is being delivered. CPR may be interrupted for up to 90 seconds when three shocks are delivered. CPR is continued between *sets* of shocks (not between individual shocks).

The steps in operation of the AED are:

1. Take infection control precautions.

2. Perform a scene size-up and initial assessment.

3. If the patient is unresponsive, nonbreathing, and pulseless, attach the defibrillator pads to the patient.

4. Turn on the power.

5. Stop CPR (if it is being performed) and clear the patient.

6. Press the button to analyze the patient's rhythm.

7. The machine will issue one of two messages: shock or no shock advised.

8. If no shock is advised, continue CPR for 1 minute and reanalyze.

9. If a shock is advised, clear the patient and press the button to deliver shock.

10. Reanalyze the rhythm.

11. Shock if advised.

12. Reanalyze the rhythm.

13. Shock if advised.

14. Check the pulse.

15. If a pulse is present, check breathing and assist ventilations as necessary.

16. If there is still no pulse, perform CPR for 1 minute and repeat the shock sequence.

When there is one rescuer present, the first step when faced with a cardiac arrest patient is to apply the AED if it is available. When two or more trained rescuers are present, one may begin CPR during defibrillator setup. Do not forget that the electric shocks are more beneficial than CPR. Do not delay defibrillation to perform CPR.

Shocks are usually given in a series of three. The pulse is not checked between the shocks but is checked before and after. If a pulse were to return between shocks, the AED would identify the heart rhythm and advise not to shock. If the first series of shocks does not cause the patient to regain a pulse, perform CPR for 1 minute and then perform a series of shocks.

Shocks are delivered using direct-current (dc) electricity. The shocks are measured in joules (J). The first shock is delivered at 200 J. The second shock is delivered at 200 to 300 J, with the final shock being delivered at 360 J. The shocks are delivered through pads placed on the chest. One pad is placed under the right clavicle and the other on the left lower ribs. The white cable goes to the right and the red goes to the left. "White to right, red to ribs" is used for remembering the placement of the pads and cables. Remember that right and left refer to the patient's right and left, not yours.

AEDs are not used on patients under 90 pounds or for children less than 12 years of age. Patients who suffer cardiac arrest from trauma rather than for medical reasons are not defibrillated. For example, motor vehicle accident patients in cardiac arrest would not be defibrillated, whereas an apparent heart attack patient would.

Patients who require defibrillation will also require advanced life support, also known as Advanced Cardiac Life Support (ACLS). This may be accomplished by paramedics on the scene and hospital emergency departments. If advanced life support is not available at the scene, it is urgent to get the patient to the emergency department.

When a patient who is defibrillated regains a pulse you will need to assess the airway carefully. Many patients regain a pulse but still require ventilation. Monitor the pulse carefully. Patients who regain a pulse can easily go back into cardiac arrest.

1. On which of the following patients would an AED be applied?
   A. An unresponsive breathing patient
   B. An unresponsive nonbreathing and pulseless patient
   C. A patient with chest pain
   D. None of the above

2. You are a First Responder who arrives alone with an automated external defibrillator on the scene of a pulseless nonbreathing patient. After your size-up and initial assessment your first action would be to:
   A. begin CPR.
   B. stand by for the EMT-Bs.
   C. apply the AED.
   D. none of the above.

3. Which of the following statements about an AED's ability to interpret cardiac rhythms is false?
   A. Correct analysis requires properly charged defibrillator batteries.
   B. AEDs will instruct the First Responder to shock ventricular fibrillation.
   C. AED cardiac rhythm analysis is only about 45% accurate.
   D. A computer microprocessor is used to analyze cardiac rhythm.

4. Which of the following procedures will help reduce the chance of accidental or inappropriate shock?
   A. Applying the AED only to unresponsive nonbreathing and pulseless patients
   B. Avoiding contact with the patient during rhythm analysis
   C. Preventing movement of monitoring leads during analysis
   D. All of the above

5. CPR may be interrupted for up to _____ seconds when delivering a series of three shocks.
   A. 30
   B. 60
   C. 90
   D. 120

6. Which of the following statements regarding AED use is true?
   A. Delivering shocks is more beneficial to the patient than is CPR.
   B. It is acceptable to delay AED use to administer oxygen.

C. AEDs can detect a pulse.

D. All of the above are true.

7. AED use is contraindicated in which of the following patients?

    A. A 120-pound 15-year-old patient

    B. A 100-pound 11-year-old patient

    C. A 95-pound 20-year-old patient

    D. A 95-pound 67-year-old patient

8. When using an AED, pulse checks are performed:

    A. before the first and after the third shock.

    B. before the first shock and after each subsequent shock.

    C. before the first shock only.

    D. by the AED, not by the First Responder.

9. After shocking a patient with the AED, you discover that the patient has a pulse. You should now:

    A. perform CPR.

    B. perform a second and third shock.

    C. check the defibrillator battery.

    D. evaluate the patient's respirations.

10. Automated defibrillation would be indicated on which of the following patients?

    A. A 13-year-old 100-pound victim who was struck by a car

    B. A 25-year-old 175-pound victim of a stabbing

    C. A 10-year-old 105-pound patient of an overdose

    D. A 65-year-old 150-pound patient who collapsed while mowing the lawn

11. The defibrillation pads are placed:

    A. over the patient's left clavicle and over the right lower ribs.

    B. just below the patient's left clavicle and over the right lower ribs.

    C. just below the patient's right clavicle and over the left lower ribs.

    D. just below the clavicle on the rescuer's right and over the lower ribs on the rescuer's left.

12. Which of the following statements is false?

    A. Patients who regain a pulse after defibrillation may require ventilation.

B. Patients who regain a pulse after defibrillation will not go back into cardiac arrest.

C. Automated defibrillators will advise a shock if ventricular fibrillation is detected.

D. Automated external defibrillator operators must memorize the treatment and defibrillation sequence.

Answers to questions 13 to 15 are based on the following scenario.

You and your partner are called to the scene of an unresponsive person. Your assessment reveals that the patient is in cardiac arrest. You have your automated external defibrillator immediately available.

13. Your next step should be to:
   A. apply the AED and analyze the rhythm.
   B. perform 1 minute of CPR.
   C. stand by for advanced life support.
   D. apply oxygen to the patient.

14. When you decide to apply the AED, you find that the batteries are dead. Your response to this situation is to:
   A. assume that the device has malfunctioned and not attempt to use it again.
   B. begin CPR while your partner replaces the battery.
   C. check the patient for a pacemaker.
   D. none of the above.

15. After delivering the second shock the machine advises you to "check pulse." This message would be given because:
   A. the patient has begun breathing.
   B. the patient has a nonshockable rhythm.
   C. the patient is in ventricular fibrillation.
   D. the AED has detected a pulse.

ANSWERS WITH RATIONALE

1. B. AEDs are applied to patients who are unresponsive, nonbreathing, and pulseless. AEDs should be brought to the side of unresponsive breathing patients and those with chest pain, but not applied unless there is an absence of pulse and respirations. This is one method of preventing inappropriate shocks.

2. C. In this scenario the AED would be applied and the rhythm analyzed immediately. Defibrillation is considered to have a greater

chance of restoring a heartbeat than CPR alone. If the AED advises not to shock, do CPR for a minute and reanalyze.

3. C. The AED is actually very accurate in cardiac rhythm analysis, making choice C false. The other statements are all true.

4. D. All of the choices listed will help prevent accidental or inappropriate shocks. By not applying a defibrillator to a patient with a pulse you cannot accidentally give a shock. Avoiding contact during rhythm analysis and not moving the cables will prevent interference and distortion of the cardiac rhythm to be analyzed.

5. C. An AED used by a trained person may be set up and three shocks delivered within 90 seconds. Since the delay is minimal, this is another reason why defibrillation must be performed before CPR.

6. A. Delivering shocks is more beneficial to the patient than is CPR. CPR will only prolong the time that the body's organs will stay alive. Defibrillation is actually a corrective measure, in that it can restore a heartbeat.

7. B. AEDs are contraindicated in patients less than 12 years of age, those weighing less than 90 pounds, and those whose heart has stopped beating from a traumatic cause (as opposed to a medical problem).

8. A. Pulse checks are performed initially and then after the third shock. There are no pulse checks between the first and second shocks and the second and third shocks. The AED analyzes the heart rhythm only. Although it will not check the pulse, it would observe any new, nonshockable heart rhythm and prompt you to check the pulse if necessary.

9. D. When you find that a patient's pulse has returned after defibrillation, the next step is to evaluate respirations. Many patients who regain a pulse do not regain respirations. Provide artificial ventilation or assist inadequate ventilations as necessary. Don't forget to monitor the pulse also. You would not provide further shocks or perform CPR on a patient with a pulse. There is no need to check the battery at this time.

10. D. The 65-year-old male has an apparent medical problem and is of an acceptable age and weight for defibrillation. The overdose patient qualifies as a medical patient, but would be ruled out since he is only 10 years old. The other patients have traumatic conditions.

11. C. The defibrillator pads are placed below the patient's right clavicle and over the left lower ribs. The pads are applied using the patient's right and left, not the First Responder's!

12. B. Choice B is false. Patients who are defibrillated successfully can easily slip back into cardiac arrest. The other choices are true. Patients who are defibrillated successfully frequently need some type of ventilatory assistance. AEDs will advise to shock V-Fib. It is vitally important that persons trained in AED use memorize the sequence and procedures.

13. A. If the AED is available and ready, apply it immediately and analyze the rhythm. This is done before oxygen, advanced life support, and CPR.

14. B. It is very important to check the AED at the beginning of every shift to prevent situations like this. They are costly to the patient and embarrassing to you. If it does happen, begin CPR while the battery is changed. Occasionally, other things happen, such as dry electrodes or missing leads. Again, begin CPR until the AED is ready.

15. B. The AED advises not to shock because the rhythm it has detected is not ventricular fibrillation or ventricular tachycardia. Any other rhythm from normal rhythms to flatline (asystole) would cause a "no shock advised" message. It is important to remember that AEDs do not check pulses or respirations. It is an important job of the operator or another trained person to monitor the patient carefully. Experienced First Responders say "treat the patient, not the machine!"

Oxygen and Supplemental Airway Information

Cognitive Objectives

At the completion of this lesson, the First Responder student will be able to:

1. Define the components of an oxygen delivery system.

2. Identify a non-rebreather face mask and state the oxygen flow requirements needed for its use.

3. Describe the indications for using a nasal cannula versus a non-rebreather face mask.

4. Identify a nasal cannula and state the flow requirements needed for its use.

5. Explain the rationale for giving basic life support artificial ventilation and airway protective skills priority over most other basic life support.

6. Explain the rationale for providing adequate oxygenation through high inspired oxygen concentrations to patients who, in the past, may have received low concentrations.

QUICK REVIEW The components of an oxygen delivery system include oxygen cylinders, pressure regulators, flowmeters, humidifiers, and oxygen delivery devices. *Oxygen cylinders* come in various sizes, the most common of which is the D or E tank. Those tanks in constant use in emergency care include:

- D cylinder: contains about 350 liters of oxygen.

- E cylinder: contains about 625 liters of oxygen.

Pressure regulators are connected to the oxygen cylinder to provide a safe working pressure of 30 to 70 psi. Cylinder pressure can be reduced in one or two steps. For a one-stop reduction, a single-stage pressure reduction is used. A two-step reduction requires a two-stage regulator. Most regulators used in emergency care are of the single-stage variety.

Flow meters allow control of the flow of oxygen in liters per minute. Connected to the pressure regulator. Most jurisdictions keep a flowmeter attached permanently to the pressure regulator.

Humidifiers are designed to be connected to a flowmeter to provide moisture to the dry oxygen coming from the supply cylinder. Dry oxygen can dehydrate the mucous membranes of a patient's airway and lungs.

Oxygen delivery devices used in the field for breathing patients include the non-rebreather mask and the nasal cannula. The *non-rebreather mask* is designed for a flow rate of 12 to 15 liters per minute and delivers approximately 80 to 90% oxygen. This is the delivery system of choice for patients with signs and symptoms of inadequate breathing and patients who are cyanotic, cool, clammy, short of breath, or suffering chest pain, suffering severe injuries, or displaying an altered mental status. The *nasal cannula* is designed for a flow rate of 1 to 6 liters per minute and delivers approximately 24 to 44% oxygen. This is the delivery system for patients who cannot tolerate a mask on the face.

The high inspired oxygen concentration of the nonrebreather mask (approximately 80 to 90%) was not routinely given to patients with chronic obstructive pulmonary diseases (COPD) such as emphysema or chronic bronchitis, or patients with black lung in the past. It was thought that since a limited number of these patients were on a secondary mechanism to breathe known as hypoxic drive, the high oxygen concentration could actually cause the patient to stop breathing. Actually, the number of COPD patients in the end stage of their disease on hypoxic drive is very limited. It makes much more sense to oxygenate the vast majority of the patients using the nonrebreather mask rather than withholding the oxygen due to fear of a very small number of patients becoming apneic. Should this actually occur, if the First Responder is watching the patient closely as he or she should be with an unstable patient, the solution is to ventilate the patient with a bag-valve-mask en route to the hospital.

The highest priority in patient treatment is airway protective skills and ventilation for basic life support. By properly opening the airway and keeping it clear of blood, secretions, and vomitus, the First Responder can prevent the patient from aspiration of foreign matter into the lungs. The need for ventilation is also a high priority to avoid patient hypoxia. That is why it is always important in the evaluation of ABCDEs to assess the breathing rate and quality.

REVIEW QUESTIONS

1. All of the following are components of an oxygen delivery system except the:
   A. pressure regulator.
   B. charcoal filter.
   C. oxygen cylinder.
   D. flowmeter.

2. When full, the D-size oxygen cylinder contains _____ liters of oxygen.
   A. 280
   B. 300
   C. 350
   D. 680

3. The pressure regulator is connected to an oxygen cylinder to provide a safe working pressure of:
   A. 5 to 30 psi.
   B. 30 to 70 psi.
   C. 75 to 90 psi.
   D. 95 to 110 psi.

4. Most regulators used in emergency care are:
   A. open filtered.
   B. two-stage.
   C. closed filtered.
   D. single-stage.

5. A device that allows control of the liters per minute of the oxygen delivery system is the:
   A. flowmeter.

B. humidifier.

C. single stage.

D. none of the above.

6. A device connected to a flowmeter to provide moisture to the dry oxygen coming from the supply cylinder is called:

   A. flowmeter.

   B. humidifier.

   C. single stage.

   D. none of the above.

7. Dry oxygen can:

   A. cause hypoxia.

   B. dehydrate the mucous membranes.

   C. increase oral secretions.

   D. increase the chance of vomiting.

8. The most common oxygen delivery device used by a First Responder is the:

   A. non-rebreather mask.

   B. nasal cannula.

   C. venturi mask.

   D. bag-valve-mask.

9. The non-rebreather mask is designed for a flow rate of _____ liters per minute.

   A. 2 to 4

   B. 6 to 10

   C. 12 to 15

   D. 16 to 20

10. The nasal cannula delivers approximately _____ % oxygen.

    A. 16 to 24

    B. 24 to 44

    C. 26 to 60

    D. none of the above.

11. The non-rebreather mask should be used on patients who are:

    A. short of breath.

    B. suffering chest pain.

    C. suffering severe injuries.

    D. all of the above.

12. The nasal cannula is designed for a flow rate of _____ liters per minute.
   A. 1 to 6
   B. 6 to 10
   C. 12 to 16
   D. none of the above

13. Examples of patients with COPD are those with:
   A. emphysema.
   B. chronic bronchitis.
   C. black lung.
   D. all of the above.

14. If a patient is on a hypoxic drive excess oxygen will:
   A. increase the breathing rate.
   B. decrease the breathing rate.
   C. be stored in the brain.
   D. cause an allergic reaction.

15. The highest priority in patient treatment is:
   A. airway protective skills.
   B. patients with fractured extremities.
   C. serious bleeding.
   D. spinal injuries.

ANSWERS WITH RATIONALE

1. B. All of the following (the pressure regulator, flowmeter, and oxygen cylinder) are components of an oxygen delivery system. The charcoal filter is part of a cigarette, not part of the delivery system.

2. C. When full, the D-size oxygen cylinder contains 350 liters of oxygen.

3. B. The pressure regulator is connected to an oxygen cylinder to provide a safe working pressure of 30 to 70 psi.

4. D. Most regulators used in emergency care are single stage.

5. A. A device that allows control of the liters per minute of the oxygen delivery system is the flowmeter. The humidifier adds moisture to the oxygen.

6. B. A device connected to a flowmeter to provide moisture to the dry oxygen coming from the supply cylinder is called a humidifier.

7. B. Dry oxygen can dehydrate the mucous membranes.

8. A. The most common oxygen delivery device used by a First Responder is the non-rebreather mask. This is because patients who are suffering from an illness or injury will benefit from oxygen. The non-rebreather provides this oxygen at a high concentration providing maximum benefit to the patient.

9. C. The non-rebreather mask is designed for a flow rate of 12–15 liters per minute. When the patient breathes in the non-rebreather bag should not collapse more than 1/3. If it collapses more than 1/3 of the way increase the oxygen flow rate.

10. B. The nasal cannula delivers approximately 24 to 44% oxygen.

11. D. The non-rebreather mask should be used on patients who are short of breath, suffering chest pain, and suffering severe injuries. These patients require the high concentration of oxygen provided by the non-rebreather.

12. A. The nasal cannula is designed for a flow rate of 1 to 6 liters per minute. When set at over 6 liters per minute, the cannula feels like a windstorm in the nose.

13. D. Examples of patients with COPD (Chronic Obstructed Pulmonary Disease) are those with emphysema, chronic bronchitis, and black lung.

14. B. When a patient has a "hypoxic drive" to breathe the brain sends a message to breathe when oxygen levels in the bloodstream are low. Administering oxygen to these patients might decrease the breathing rate because the brain senses enough oxygen and feels it is not necessary to breathe. Oxygen will not cause an allergic reaction. It is important to remember that even patients who have the hypoxic drive can become seriously ill and injured. When this is the case administer oxygen with a non-rebreather and monitor the patient's breathing carefully.

15. A. The highest priority in patient treatment is airway protective skills, then ventilation, then bleeding control, then mental status and spinal injuries.

Medical Emergencies
(Supplemental Information)

Cognitive Objectives

At the completion of this lesson, the First Responder student will be able to:

1.   Discuss coronary artery disease and its complications (angina, AMI, CHF).

2.   Discuss patient assessment findings of a patient with cardiac compromise.

3.   Describe the emergency medical care of the cardiac compromise patient.

4.   Define diabetes, insulin, glucose, and hypoglycemia.

5.   State the steps in the emergency medical care of the patient taking diabetic medicine with an altered mental status and a history of diabetes.

6.   Establish the relationship between airway management and the patient with altered mental status.

7.   List causes of allergic reactions.

8.   Recognize the patient experiencing an anaphylactic reaction.

9.   Describe the emergency medical care of a patient with anaphylaxis.

10. Establish the relationship between a patient with an allergic reaction and airway management.

11. Differentiate between the general category of patients having an allergic reaction and patients having an allergic reaction requiring immediate medical care.

12. List four ways that poisons enter the body.

13. List signs and symptoms associated with poisoning.

14. Discuss the assessment of a patient who has ingested a poison.

15. Describe the steps in the emergency medical care of a patient who ingested a poison.

16. Establish the relationship between a patient suffering from poisoning or overdose and airway management.

17. List the assessment findings of an injected poisoning from an insect bite and/or sting.

18. Discuss the emergency medical care of bites and stings.

19. Recognize the problems that patients experience from water-related emergencies.

20. Describe the complications of near-drowning.

QUICK REVIEW Although the First Responder treats all patients with signs and symptoms of cardiac compromise in the same manner as discussed later in this section, there is no need for the First Responder to diagnose what kind of heart problem the patient may be having. It is useful to have some background knowledge of the most common cardiovascular disorders: coronary artery disease, angina pectoris, acute myocardial infarction, and congestive heart failure.

Diseases affect the arteries of the heart, often causing a narrowing or blockage from depositing cholesterol plaques on the interior wall of the arteries. This process is commonly called *coronary artery disease* (CAD). The factors that put a person at risk of developing CAD are heredity, age, hypertension or high blood pressure, obesity, lack of exercise, elevated blood levels of cholesterol and triglycerides, and cigarette smoking.

Angina pectoris means, literally, a pain in the chest. CAD has caused a narrowing of the coronary arteries. Under stress or exertion, when the heart needs more oxygenated blood, an inadequate supply makes it to portions of the heart muscle. This oxygen-starved tissue causes chest pain. Since the pain of angina pectoris comes on after stress or exertion, frequently it diminishes once the patient rests for awhile. Seldom does this painful attack last longer than 3 to 5 minutes.

Patients being treated by a physician for angina usually carry a medication called *nitroglycerin,* which is dissolved under their tongue when they get chest pain. The nitro is used to enlarge or dilate the coronary arteries temporarily to let more oxygenated blood pass through. The typical physician order for an angina patient when they get chest pain from stress or exertion is to rest and take up to three nitros, one at a time, over a 10-minute period. If the pain is not relieved, they should call an ambulance since they may actually be experiencing an acute myocardial infarction (AMI) or heart attack.

The condition in which a portion of the myocardium dies as a result of oxygen starvation is called an *AMI* or *heart attack*. AMI is brought on by the narrowing or occlusion (blockage) of a coronary artery. There are over 1 million cases of AMI each year in the United States alone. A major portion of these cases result in sudden death, which is defined as a cardiac arrest that occurs within 2 hours of the onset of symptoms.

Congestive heart failure (CHF) is a condition of excessive fluid buildup in the lungs and/or other organs and body parts. The fluid buildup causes edema, or swelling. The disorder is termed *congestive* because fluids congest or clog the organs. It is termed *heart failure* because the congestion both results from and aggravates failure of the heart to function properly. The congestion may also result from and aggravate failure of the lungs to function properly.

Assessment of a patient with cardiac compromise includes performing the initial assessment, performing a focused history and physical exam, inquiring about onset, provocation, quality, radiation, severity and time, obtaining a SAMPLE history, and taking baseline vital signs.

The signs and symptoms associated with cardiac compromise include:

- Pain, pressure, or discomfort in the chest or upper abdomen (epigastrium)

- Difficulty breathing

- Palpitations

- Sudden onset of sweating with nausea or vomiting

- Anxiety (feeling of impending doom, irritability)

- Abnormal pulse

- Abnormal blood pressure

The emergency care steps for a patient experiencing cardiac compromise include:

1. Place the patient in the position of comfort, which is usually sitting up to ease breathing. If hypotensive, the patient may feel better lying down.

2. Apply high-concentration oxygen through a non-rebreather mask.

3. Prepare the patient for prompt transport, especially if the patient has:
   a. No history of cardiac problems.
   b. A history of cardiac problems but does not have nitroglycerin.
   c. A systolic BP of less than 100.

4. The EMT-Bs on the ambulance may have a local protocol to assist the patient with nitro.

Glucose is a form of sugar that is the body's basic source of energy. The sugars that we eat are converted into glucose and then absorbed into the bloodstream. For sugars to enter the cells, insulin, a hormone produced by the pancreas, must be present. The condition brought about by decreased insulin production is know as diabetes mellitus. These patients have too much sugar, which cannot enter the cells due to insufficient or absent insulin. The most common medical emergency for the diabetic is hypoglycemia, or low blood sugar. Hypoglycemia is caused when the diabetic:

- Takes too much insulin, thereby putting too much sugar into the cells and leaving too little sugar in the blood

- Reduces sugar intake by not eating

- Overexercises or overexerts himself, thus using sugars faster than normally

- Vomits a meal, emptying the stomach of sugar as well as other food

Prehospital treatment of the diabetic depends on rapid identification of the patient with an altered mental status and a history of diabetes. The following signs and symptoms are associated with a diabetic:

1. Rapid onset of altered mental status
   a. After missing a meal on a day prescribed insulin was taken
   b. After vomiting a meal on a day prescribed insulin was taken
   c. After an unusual amount of physical exercise or work
   d. May occur with no identifiable predisposing factor

2. Intoxicated appearance, staggering, slurred speech, to complete unresponsiveness

3. Elevated heart rate

4. Cold, clammy skin

5. Hunger

6. Seizures

7. Insulin or an oral medication used to treat diabetes found in refrigerator or at the scene

8. Uncharacteristic behavior

9. Anxiety

10. Combativeness

Steps in the management of a diabetic emergency include the following:

1. Give oral glucose in accordance with local protocol if the patient has a history of diabetes, has an altered mental status and is awake enough to swallow. This can be done using a tongue depressor with glucose paste placed between the teeth and gum.

2. Reassess the patient. If he or she loses the ability to swallow, remove the tongue depressor.

It is important to watch the airway of a patient with an altered level of consciousness as he or she may not be able to swallow secretions or can vomit and aspirate if there is no gag reflex.

The First Responder should be able to recognize a patient experiencing an allergic reaction. This patient has an exaggerated response of the body's immune system. This response can range from a minor irritation to a severe life-threatening condition known as anaphylaxis. In a minor allergic reaction there may be swelling, hives, and itching or watery eyes. In anaphylaxis, exposure to an allergen will cause blood vessels to dilate rapidly and cause a drop in blood pressure. Many tissues may swell, including those in the respiratory system. This swelling can obstruct the airway. The lower airways can constrict causing wheezing. They may also have a decreased mental status, hoarseness, and/or stridor. Causes of allergic reactions include:

- Insect stings

- Foods such as nuts, eggs, milk, or shellfish

- Plants

- Medications

- Dust, chemicals, soaps, and so on

The emergency care steps for anaphylaxis include:

1. Give high-concentration oxygen and evaluate the need for bag-valve-mask ventilation.

2. Call for immediate EMS response, as EMT-Bs are trained to administer a prescribed epinephrine autoinjector under medical control, which may be lifesaving.

3. Treat for shock and prepare for immediate transport.

The important lesson to remember here is that there is a relationship between airway maintenance and a severe allergic reaction in that the airway can swell and become totally occluded. The First Responder needs to be able to differentiate between an allergic reaction and anaphalaxis based on the presence of respiratory distress, wheezing, airway swelling and hypotension.

Poisons are substances that can harm the body sometimes seriously enough to create a medical emergency. Poisons are classified into four types according to how they enter the body: ingested, inhaled, absorbed, and injected. When conducting a patient assessment of a patient suspected of having ingested a poison, the First Responder should consider the following questions:

- What substance was involved?

- When did the exposure occur?

- How much was ingested?

- Over how long a period of time did the ingestion occur?

- What interventions have the patient's family or well-meaning bystanders taken?

- What is the patient's estimated weight?

- What effects is the patient experiencing from the ingestion?

The emergency medical care for an ingested poison includes:

1. Detect and treat immediately life-threatening problems with the initial assessment.

2. Perform a First Responder patient assessment, including a SAMPLE history.

3. Assess baseline vital signs.

4. Consult medical direction personnel or contact poison control personnel for the use of activated charcoal following your local treatment protocol.

5. Make sure that the transporting ambulance takes all containers, bottles, and labels of the substance in question.

It is important for the First Responder to remember that poisons or overdoses can lead to an altered mental status, which in turn will decrease the patient's ability to protect the airway. That is why the First Responder has a very important role in maintaining the airway and preventing aspiration if the patient vomits.

The assessment findings of insect bites and stings include:

- Altered states of awareness

- Noticeable stings or bites on the skin

- Puncture marks, especially on the fingers, forearms, toes, and legs

- Blotchy or mottled skin

- Localized pain or itching

- Numbness in a limb or body part

- Burning sensations at the site, followed by pain spreading throughout the limb

- Redness

- Swelling or blistering at the site

- Weakness or collapse

- Difficult breathing and abnormal pulse rate

- Headache and dizziness

- Chills and fever

- Nausea and vomiting

- Muscle cramps, chest tightening, and joint pains

- Excessive saliva formation and profuse sweating

- Anaphylaxis

The First Responder should provide emergency care for injected toxins to include:

1. Treat for hyperfusion or shock.

2. Call medical direction for advice.

3. Do not pull out a bee or wasp stinger and venom sac, as you may actually squeeze more venom into the patient.

4. Remove jewelry from affected limbs.

5. If local protocol permits and the wound is an extremity, place constricting bands above and below the sting or bite site.

6. Keep the limb immobilized and the patient still to prevent distribution of the poison to other parts of the body.

The First Responder should look for the following problems in water-related accident victims:

- Airway obstruction

- Cardiac arrest

- Signs of heart attack

- Injuries to the head and neck

- Internal injuries

- Generalized cooling or hypothermia

- Substance abuse

- Drowning or near-drowning (the complications of near-drowning can include: spinal injury, a nonbreathing patient, gastric distension, or hypothermia)

REVIEW QUESTIONS

1. Complications of coronary artery disease may include:
   A. angina.
   B. AMI.
   C. congestive heart failure.
   D. all of the above.

2. The factors that put a person at risk of developing coronary artery disease include all of the following except:
   A. elevated cholesterol.
   B. hypotension.
   C. cigarette smoking.
   D. lack of exercise.

3. To treat a patient experiencing cardiac compromise, the First Responder should:
   A. administer nitro to the patient.
   B. place the patient in a position of comfort.
   C. apply a nasal cannula.
   D. all of the above.

4. The assessment findings of a patient with cardiac compromise may include:
   A. palpitations.
   B. feeling of impending doom.
   C. abnormal blood pressure.
   D. any of the above.

5. For sugar to enter the cells, the body must have:
   A. glycogen.
   B. insulin.
   C. exercise.
   D. glucose.

6. Hypoglycemia is caused when the diabetic:
   A. forgets to take his or her insulin.
   B. skips his or her exercise routine for a day.
   C. reduces sugar intake by not eating.
   D. overeats on fats and carbohydrates.

7. A diabetic emergency may include which of the following signs and symptoms?
   A. cold, clammy skin
   B. hunger and elevated heart rate
   C. anxiety and combativeness
   D. all of the above

8. When a patient has an altered level of consciousness, a primary concern of the First Responder should be to:
   A. place a pillow under the patient's head.
   B. position the airway properly if there is no gag reflex.
   C. give the patient liquid sugar to drink.
   D. none of the above.

9. An allergic reaction is defined as:
   A. an exaggerated response by the body's immune system.
   B. swollen tissue, causing complete airway obstruction.
   C. hypotension and increased intracerebral pressure.
   D. none of the above.

10. Causes of allergic reactions include:
    A. peanuts and medications.
    B. foods such as nuts, eggs, milk, and shellfish.
    C. dust, chemicals, and soaps.
    D. all of the above.

11. Anaphylaxis is defined as:
    A. hives and itching from an allergic reaction.
    B. local swelling.
    C. cardiovascular collapse as a result of allergic reaction.
    D. all of the above.

12. Why is airway management a concern in an allergic reaction?
    A. The patient may develop hives.
    B. The lower airways begin to wheeze.
    C. The airway may swell up.
    D. None of the above.

13. Of the following, which is not a way that poisons enter the body?
    A. Ingestion
    B. Defecation
    C. Absorption
    D. Injection

14. Typical signs and symptoms associated with a poisoning include:
    A. altered mental status.
    B. abnormal pulse rate.
    C. difficulty breathing.
    D. any of the above.

15. When assessing a patient with a suspected poisoning by ingestion, be sure to ask:
    A. the patient's weight.
    B. where the substance was purchased.
    C. if the patient has any recent injuries.
    D. if someone was watching the patient ingest the materials.

16. When consulting with medical control after evaluating a poisoning victim, you may be asked to give the patient:
    A. spirits of ipecac.
    B. sugar under the tongue.
    C. activated charcoal.
    D. all of the above.

17. If the patient is getting groggy and sleepy when you begin to treat him or her for a suspected poisoning you should:
    A. quickly administer activated charcoal to the patient.
    B. watch the airway very closely to prevent aspiration of vomitus.
    C. tell him or her to stay awake.
    D. apply cold packs in the groin.

18. Assessment findings from an insect bite or sting may include any of the following except:
    A. numbness in a limb or body part.
    B. blotchy or mottled skin.
    C. a pulsatile mass in the patient's abdomen.
    D. swelling or blistering at the site.

19. Emergency medical care for an injected toxin includes:
    A. pulling out the wasp stinger.
    B. placing a tourniquet above and below the bite site.
    C. immobilizing the injured extremity.
    D. all of the above.

20. Complications of near-drowning may include:
    A. head injury.
    B. spine injury.
    C. airway compromise.
    D. all of the above.

ANSWERS WITH RATIONALE

1. D. Complications of coronary artery disease may include angina, AMI, and congestive heart failure.

2. B. The factors that put a person at risk of developing coronary artery disease include elevated cholesterol, hypertension, cigarette smoking, and lack of exercise. Hypotension is low blood pressure and is not a factor for this disease.

3. B. To treat a patient experiencing cardiac compromise, the First Responder should place the patient in the position of comfort. A non-rebreather mask is used for oxygen administration, and nitro is given by the EMT-B, not the First Responder.

4. D. The assessment findings of a patient with a cardiac compromise may include palpitations, the feeling of impending doom, and abnormal blood pressure.

5. B. For sugar to enter the cells, the body must have insulin. The form of sugar used by the body is called glucose.

6. C. Hypoglycemia is caused when the diabetic reduces sugar intake by not eating. Diabetic coma or hyperglycemia could be caused by forgetting to take insulin, skipping the exercise routine for the day, or by overeating fats and carbohydrates.

7. D. A diabetic emergency may include the following signs and symptoms: cold, clammy skin, hunger and elevated heart rate, and anxiety and combativeness.

8. B. When a patient has an altered level of consciousness, a primary concern of the First Responder should be to position the airway

properly if there is no gag reflex. Patients with an altered level of consciousness should not be given anything by mouth, for fear of vomiting and aspiration. In patients with an altered level of consciousness, placing pillow under the patient's head will cause the airway to close.

9. A. An allergic reaction is defined as an exaggerated response by the body's immune system. This may range from hives and itching to anaphylaxis, which is a serious medical emergency.

10. D. Causes of allergic reactions include peanuts and medications, foods such as nuts, eggs, milk, and shellfish, and dust, chemicals, and soaps.

11. C. Anaphylaxis is defined as cardiovascular collapse as a result of an exaggerated immune response. The reverse is not always true; that is, not all cardiac collapse is anaphalaxis. A minor allergic reaction can show local swelling and hives.

12. C. Airway management is a concern in an allergic reaction because the airway may swell up and occlude.

13. B. Defication is a way that poisons exit the body. The other choices represent ways that poisons enter the body.

14. D. Typical signs and symptoms associated with poisoning include altered mental status, abnormal pulse rate, and difficulty breathing.

15. A. When assessing a patient with a suspected poisoning by ingestion, be sure to ask the patient's weight. This is important to medical control and the emergency department, as the lighter the patient, the less poison it takes to kill them.

16. C. When consulting with medical control personnel after evaluating a poisoning victim, you may be asked to give the patient activated charcoal. Syrup of ipecac (not spirits of ipecac) is rarely used in the field.

17. B. If the patient is getting groggy and sleepy when you begin to treat him or her for a suspected poisoning, you should watch the airway very closely to prevent aspiration of vomitus. Do not rush to administer anything by mouth to a patient whose level of consciousness is diminishing. Cold packs in the groin is a street cure that doesn't work.

18. C. Assessment findings from an insect bite or sting may include numbness in a limb or body part, blotchy or mottled skin,

and swelling or blistering at the site. A pulsatile mass in the patient's abdomen is a sign of an abdominal aortic aneurysm.

19. C. Emergency medical care for an injected toxin includes immobilizing the injured extremity. If a device is applied to the extremity, it is a constricting venous band approved by medical control. Do not pull out the stinger, as you may squeeze more toxin into the patient.

20. D. Complications of near-drowning may include head injury, spine injury, and airway compromise.